BOSU FITNESS

Marina Aagaard

BOSU FITNESS

Complete cardio, strength and core conditioning

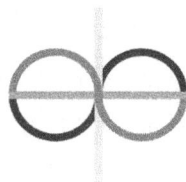

aagaard

BOSU FITNESS
Complete cardio, strength and core conditioning

First Edition

ISBN: 978-87-92693-70-9

Photos:	Claus Petersen, CPhotography, 16, 19.
	Marina Aagaard, 8, 10, 14, 17, 24, 29, 30, 32, 33, 40, 42, 46, 69, 82, 84, 86, 88, 92, 94, 96, 98, 100, 102, 112.
	Exercise model: Diploma coach and chef *Morten Kirstein*.
	Henrik Elstrup, 86, 90, 100, 102, 104, 106.
	istock © side: 12-13 © cc-stock, 38, 48 © Catherine Yeulet, 50 © Suprijono Suharjoto, 61, 62, 80 © Eliza Snow.
	sxc.hu © side: 66 © Matúš Petrila.
	microsoft clipart: 22, 108.
Cover photo:	istock © Rich Legg
Portrait p. 126:	Henrik Jern
Text and drawings:	Marina Aagaard
Printed:	Lulu, USA, 2013

No book can replace the services of a physician, exercise physiologist or other qualified health or exercise professionel. The programs and exercises in this book may not be for everyone. Any application of the information set forth in the following pages is at the reader's discretion and sole risk.

Marina Aagaard
www.fitnesswellnessworld.com

PREFACE

BOSU FITNESS is a comprehensive guide to designing fun and effective workouts using the BOSU Balance Trainer.

The BOSU was introduced in 2000 and has since become a popular part of fitness classes around the world.
Many fitness centres have one or more BOSU's in their gym for balance and stability work and the BOSU is also a versatile piece of equipment for group exercise for either cardio, resistance training or hybrid workouts.

This book has been written to provide program and exercise inspiration for physical trainers, personal trainers, group exercise instructors and physio-therapists using the BOSU for various types of training in different formats. The primary goal is to provide an overview over the numerous exercises and novel ideas for complete program design, format and sequencing.

Some unique features of this book:

1. A table of base moves for cardio variation.
2. Multiple ideas, 'templates', for strength and circuit classes.
3. Two complete BOSU group exercise workouts choreographed to music. Also for use in one-on-one training.

It is my hope that this book will provide inspiration for more workouts and more motivating workouts with the BOSU.

Marina Aagaard, MFE
Aarhus, 2013

TABLE OF CONTENTS

TABLE OF CONTENTS

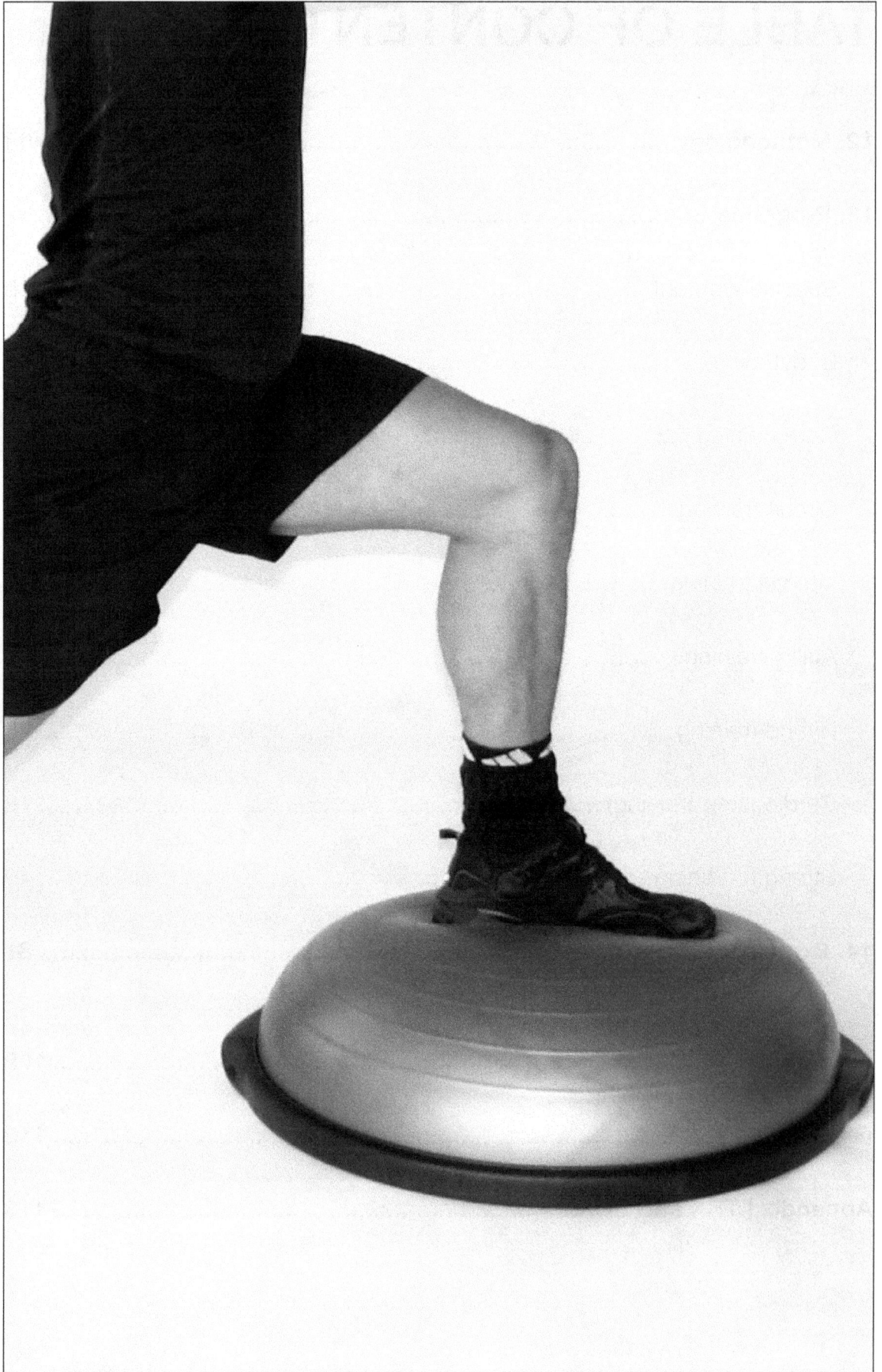

TABLE OF CONTENT

CHAPTER 1 | INTRODUCTION

The BOSU Balance Trainer, then and now a popular piece of fitness equipment, was launched in 2000 by inventor David Weck, USA.

The BOSU is an inflatable dome on a solid platform. It measures 62,5 cm, 25 inches, in diameter, with a height of 20-25 cm, 8-10 inches. The weight is 7 kg.

The unstable surface is excellent for training stability and balance in strength training as well as cardio workouts; the BOSU can be used as a fun and challenging 'step'.

The BOSU is a versatile piece of equipment, great for personal training as well as group exercise.

The name BOSU was an acronym for BOth Sides Up, later changed to BOth Sides Utilized. Meaning that not only can you use either side of the BOSU, but BOSU training also *represents an approach to exercise that is more mindful than traditional training"* (BOSU, 2006).

BOSU training is quite demanding and requires your full attention and concentration.
However, BOSU training can easily be adapted for enjoyable workouts for most target groups.

Enjoy.

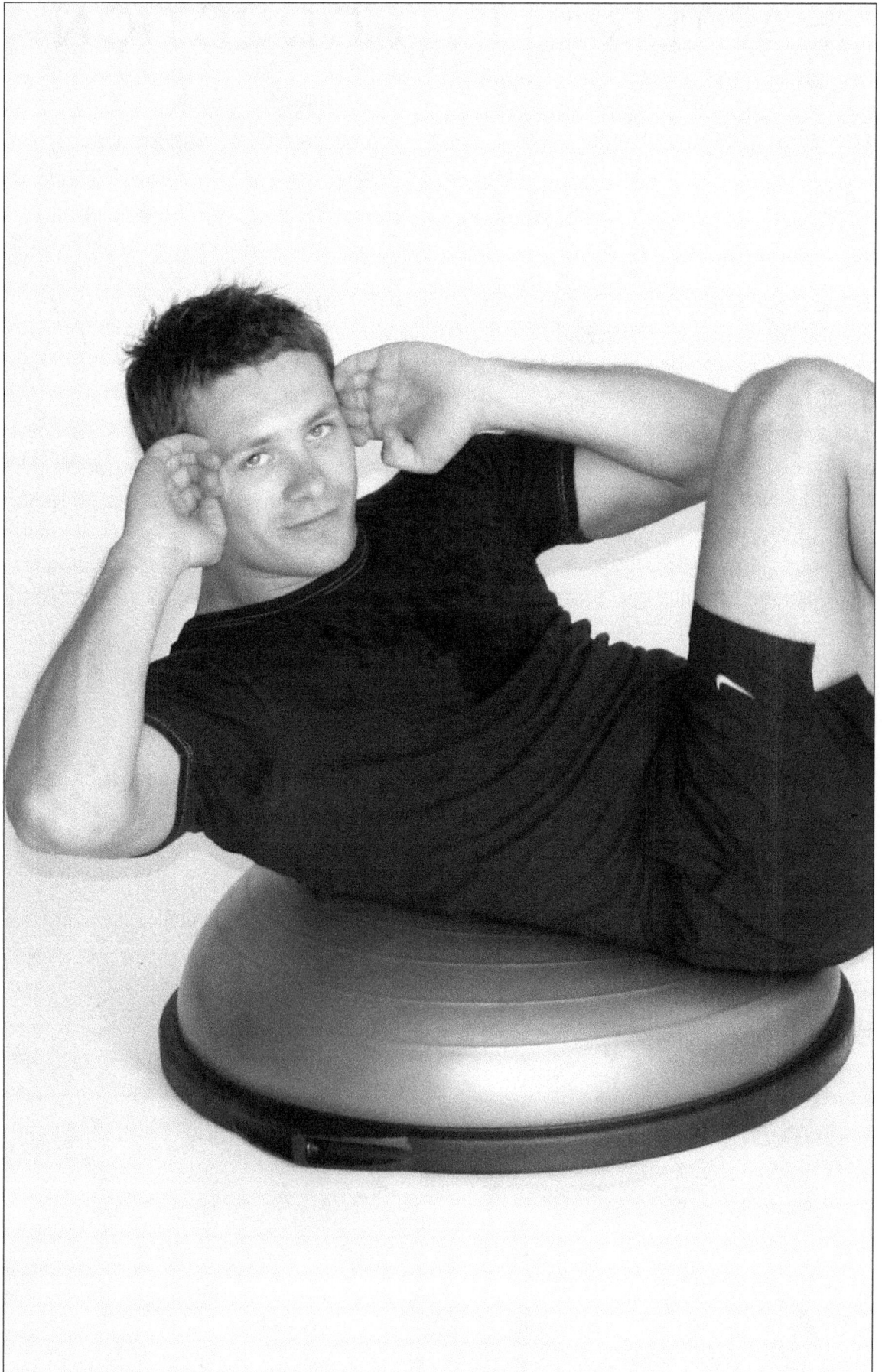

CHAPTER 2 | **BOSU BASICS**

BOSU ADVANTAGES

There is a number of advantages to working out with the BOSU:

- The BOSU can be used on either side: On the dome side, top side, or the platform side, under side, as a large 'rocking board'.

- The unstable top, dome, means that in most exercises you have to stabilize; you improve strength *and* stability and balance.

- To keep your balance, you need to maintain an upright and stable posture by activiting your core, a.o. transversus abdominis and mm. multifidii. This way you get an excellent postural workout.

- The curvature of the dome means, that when you are prone or supine on the dome, there is a larger range of motion in many strength and flexiility exercises.

- The BOSU is a soft, comfortable and versatile workout 'bench'.

- It is an excellent all-round piece of equipment for balance, toning and cardio work as well as agility workouts with hops and jumps.

- The BOSU is an obvious choice for circuit training; at one or more stations or organized in rows for fun exercises and games for children and adults alike.

- The BOSU increases your body-consciousness; during workouts one can clearly feel the muscles working together to stabilize.

- The price is very reasonable compared to the numerous applications.
  However, the price may also be the limiting factor, when considering buying BOSU's for group exercise for 20-50 people.

The only disadvantage is that the BOSU is rather heavy; not that easy to move around or carry with you; e.g. it is not suited for travel use.

Space requirements for BOSU is about 12-16 square feet (3-4 kvm.) with space for stepping safely on and off the BOSU in all directions – with a safe distance to the walls and other equipment or 'obstacles'.
The exerciser(s) should be able to lie in a prone or supine position on the BOSU without touching anyone with the hands or feet.

INFLATABLE EQUIPMENT

The BOSU Stability Trainer was the first of its kind in 2000. Since then it has been improved upon and also similar products have emerged.

There are also smaller inflatable balance equipment, eg. AeroStep and AirDisc.
These are also recommended for varying stability training programs. However, they do not offer quite as many options as the BOSU (dome).

Note: Use instability training wisely; sensible progressions and programs, so that you improve – not diminish – stability and sports performance. Include stable surface stability work.

INFLATING THE BOSU

When buying a BOSU you should first read the manual to ensure, that you handle and inflate it correctly for optimal performance.

Maximum dome height is approximately 20-25 cm, 8-10 inches.

The surface should feel firm with a sligth give to it.

Note: Recommended inflation level, dome height, must not be exceeded.

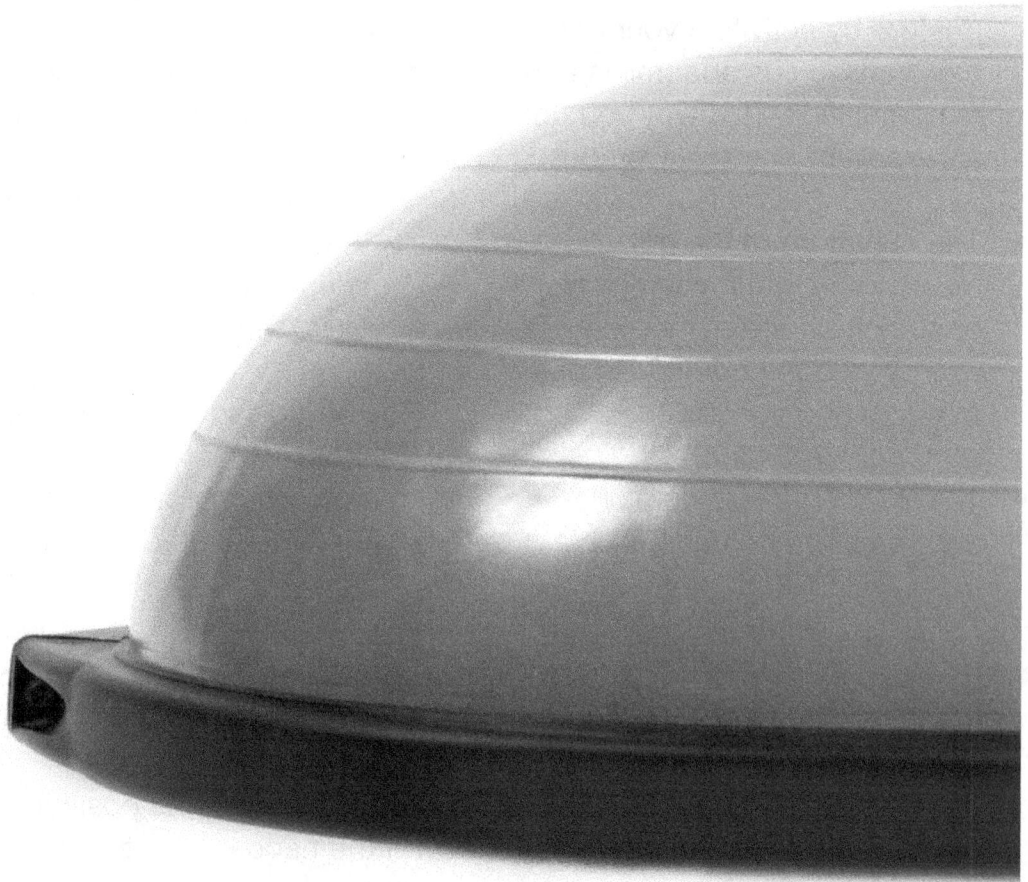

HANDLING AND STORAGE

Handle your BOSU with care to increase performance and durability:

- Keep it clean, no dust, sand or other impurities.

- The surface, floor or mat, should be dry and clean.

- Avoid scratching or puncturing the dome surface with zippers or buckles.
  Preferably take off sharp jewellery or watches before workouts.

- Wear indoor footwear or bare feet. Wipe off the soles of your shoes, so that pebbles, glass and other debris is removed, before you step onto the BOSU.

- Storage in strong heat or cold may affect the BOSU.
  Avoid direct sunlight and do not place it close to heaters.

- The BOSU can be cleaned with a moist cloth. Use warm water or a mild soap.
  Avoid all kinds of strong cleaning agents solvents and scouring powders.

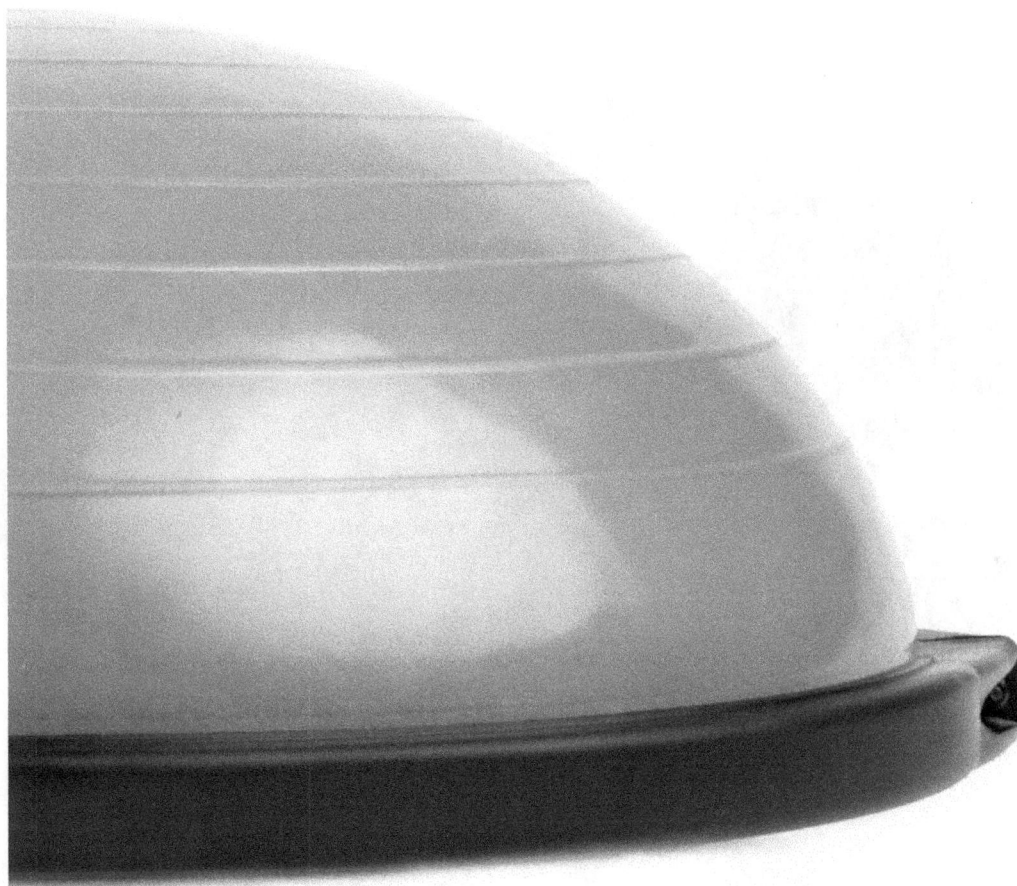

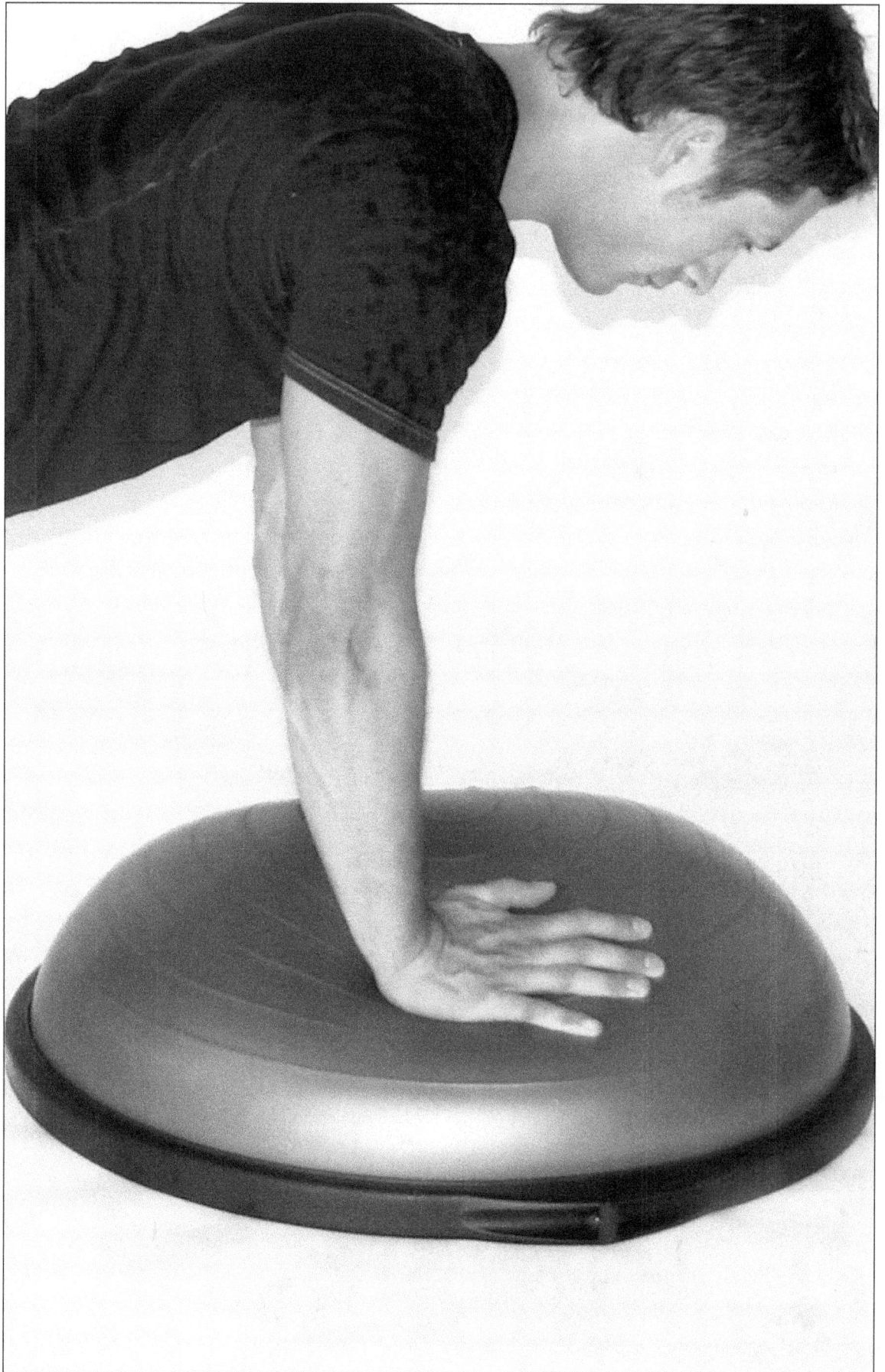

CHAPTER 3 | **TECHNIQUE**

The exercises are initiated by a strong and stable starting position:

Upright and strong with stable core, mid-section.
For extra stability during demanding exercises; focus on contracting the pelvic floor and the transversus abdominis as needed.

The shoulder blades should be 'in place' during e.g. planks and push-ups; keep the shoulder girdle stable.

Avoid poor posture during workouts; avoid that 1) the head and shoulders drop, 2) the lumbar spine hyperextends unnaturally and 3) knees and elbows hyperextend.

During planks, you should observe that head, shoulder blades and spine are all in a neutral position, so the body is in a 'straight line'.

Note: Strengthen your wrists gradually to avoid overuse injury.

A strong and stable posture and correct exercise technique will enhance the workout, improve the results and provide a solid base for better future workouts.

Depending on the exercise, whether it is an isolation exercise or complex exercise, the exercise focus is either on a few primary muscles or many muscles working together.

Observe gradual progression. Start exercises at the easiest level and do not move on to the next level before mastering the previous levels.
If you do, you risk 'programming' a faulty and inefficient motor pattern, which is difficult to reverse.

Trainers need to differentiate their chosen exercises, so every exercise fits the person or target group.

Exercisers need to listen to the body, go at their own pace and take a rest or modify exercises, when necessary.

Breathing should be deep, even and natural; exhale, when the muscle shortens, concentric contraction, and inhale, when the muscles elongates, eccentric action. Inhale through the nose, exhale through the mouth. During isometric exercises: Keep breathing, do not hold your breath.

STARTING POSITION

Before the workout make a quick posture check:

From the front imagine a plumb line through the center of the body. Around this line the body, shoulders and hips, forms a symmetrical image; if you have mirrors, you can use them.

From the side imagine a plumb line passing through the ear, shoulder, hip, knee and ankle.

If you see a major deviation or problem, it may need to be corrected by you (or a physiotherapist), before starting the workout.

Focus points for the starting position standing on the floor:

- Feet hip-width apart.
- Feet forward or slight outward.
- Feet firmly on the ground with even weight distribution.
- Knees aligned with feet.
- Knees relaxed, not locked, not bent.
- Contract the pelvic floor muscles and transversus abdominis – for practice (then relax).
- Pelvis in neutral position.
- Spine in neutral position, normal lordosis.
- Shoulderblades in neutral.
- Shoulders level and lowered.
- Neck in neutral position.
- Tongue in resting position in the roof of the mouth behind the front teeth.

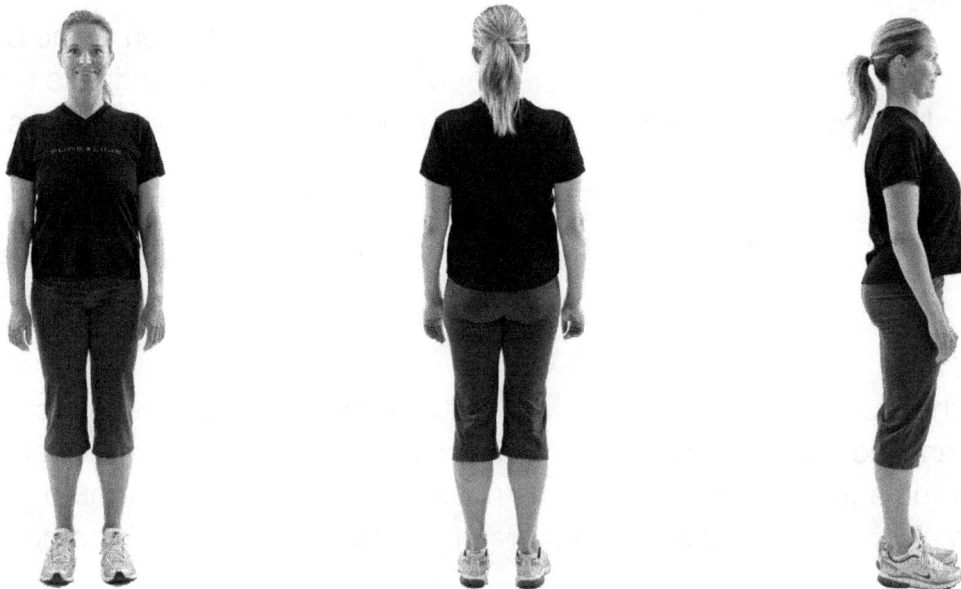

STARTING POSITION ON THE BOSU

Standing
Standing on the dome can be quite challenging: This is excellent for balance and stabilization workouts.

Stand tall with and erect posture and concentrate, otherwise you will loose your balance.
Start with your feet shoulder-width apart. Then hip-width apart and then together and on one leg only. Choose position according to the goal of the exercise.

Focus points standing on the BOSU:

- Foot/feet as stable as possible
- Toes forward
- Foot/feet in neutral position
- Avoid plantar- and dorsiflexion
- Avoid inversion and eversion
- Upright posture – focus
- Avoid locking the knees
- Maintain core control and control the movements.

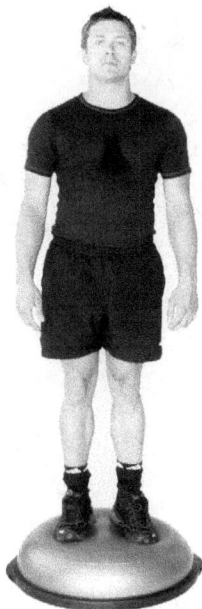

Kneeling
Many different positions and points of support on the BOSU or the floor.

On all fours
Different positions with different points of suppont on the BOSU or the floor to stabilize.

Sitting
The BOSU is low, so the seated position may not be comfortable; you need to put your legs in a suitable position. Keep the torso erect with a nice posture.

Supine and bridge position
Position the torso, arms and legs according to the exercise.
Feet on the floor.
The BOSU, dome, is comfortable; it is soft and follows the curve of the back. And you are in a stable position (it's not like being on a big ball), when the feet are on the floor.

Sidelying
Position the torso and arms according to the exercise.
Keep the neck in neutral position.
Feet can be staggered on the floor, on top of one another or off the floor.

Prone
Position the torso and arms according to the exercise.
Neck in neutral position. Toes or lower legs on (or off) the floor.
Note.: When supine, the limb range of motion (downward) is limited.

CORE TRAINING

The core is the center of the body; all the muscles between the diaphragm and the pelvic floor, including the deep stabilizing muscles; *the core*, hence the name **core training**.
Core training is import, because a strong core, center of the body, provides stability and improves force transfer from the lower body, legs, to the upper body.
Core training in some form should always be a part of basic training.

The core includes:

m. transversus abdominis; you can feel this muscle, when you laugh or when you cough, and the small deep back muscles, *mm. multifidii.*

Core training involves these and other 'inner unit' muscles, small stabilizing back muscles and the m. quadratus lumborum and the pelvic floor, and the 'outer unit' muscles, abdominal and back muscles.

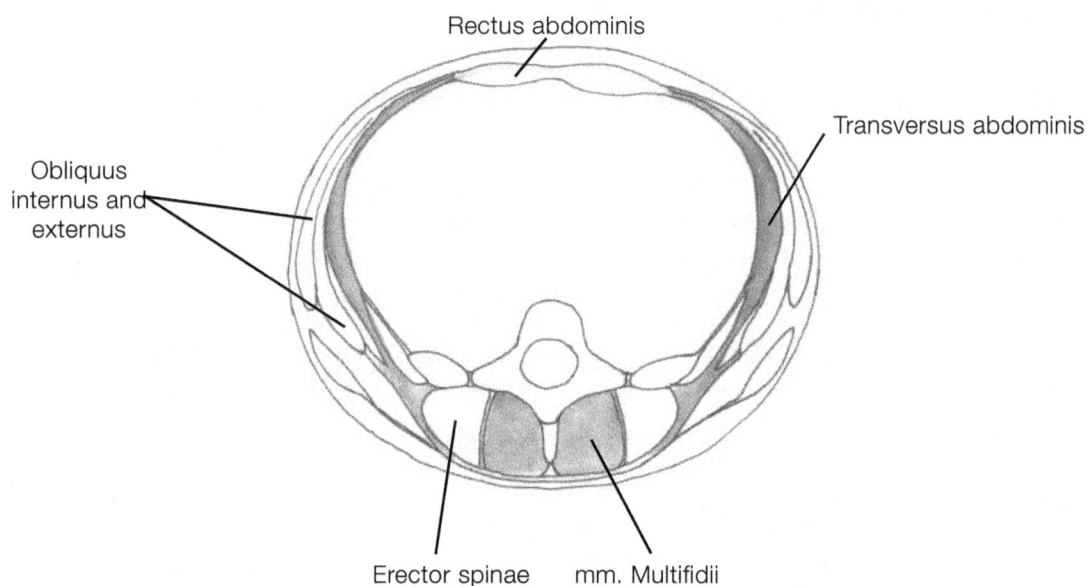

Rectus abdominis

Transversus abdominis

Obliquus internus and externus

Erector spinae   mm. Multifidii

Cross section of the torso. Spine, at the back (bottom of drawing) and around the torso the abdominal muscles in layers on top of each other. Transversus abdomins and the back stabilizer muscles mm. multifidii are indicated with a dark colour.

As a rehearsel for training your core, you can practice activating the transversus abdominis:

- Think of the abdominal region as a clock, with '12 o'clock' by the sternum, '6 o'clock by the pubic bone, and '3 and 9 o'clock at the sides of the torso.

- Put hands at waist level on each side of the navel with the middle fingers pointing to each other.

- Think of drawing '3 and 9 o'clock' on the clock together, in towards the navel;

- The transversus abdominis is contracted; the hands slide towards each other and the middle fingers touch.

This method can assist you in 'locating' and contracting your transversus abdomins, TA, when extra stability is needed.

Tip: If you put your hands on your lower back, you should also be able to feel the TA contracting.

The ability to maintain neutral posture in the spine, can be checked with an easy test performed supine on the floor:

In supine position lift your legs to a table-top position, 90 degree angle at the hips, while contracting the core, a.o. the rectus abdominis and the transversus abdominis.

Beginners can keep the knee bent at a 90 degree angle – and keep the low back on the floor.

Advanced exercisers can have the legs straight, vertical, and maintain natural lordosis (you can put a finger under the low back, not the hand).

One or both legs are lowered towards the floor with the aim of touching the foot/feet to the floor.

If the back starts hyperextending during this test, it indicates insufficient abdominal, core, control.

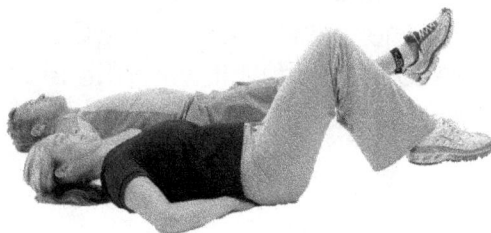

TRAINING TECHNIQUE

Optimal training technique depends on knowledge about the exercise and

- Controlled movements
- Correct lifting technique
- Full range of motion
- Exercise execution

Controlled movements
The muscles must contract and act with control, you need to control the movement concentrically as well as eccentrically and with flow in each repetition and set; smooth, identical movements without pausing in the 'top' or 'bottom' of the exercise; the end ranges of motion.

Correct lifting technique
Correct lifting technique is lifting with a good posture and the right technique for a given exercise as well as carrying equipment:

Get close to the BOSU, stand firmly and lift the BOSU with control, watch the wrists. Carry the BOSU close to the body. Lift with the legs and arms, not just the back.

Full range of motion
The amplitude of the exercise, *range of motion (ROM)* depends on the joint structure and tissues

The muscles should be trained in a full, natural, range of motion with a suitable load for that muscle. Meaning that the muscles should be trained in their full range of motion, while keeping in mind, that some positions, end ranges of motion, are not suited for maximal external load.

Example:
The arm can be moved well behind the torso in preparation for a hand-ball throw (the ball weighs 325-475 grams), but the same range of motion is potentially harmful with a very large external load, like a barbell with heavy plates in a benchpress.

Exercise execution
A safe and effective exercise execution begins with a good posture; neck, spine, shoulderblades and pelvis in neutral position and elbows and knees in a natural (straight), but not 'locked', position.

SAFETY PRECAUTIONS

Proceed with caution, be patient, learn the technique.
Take classes from a proficient BOSU trainer the first couple of times.

General focus points for safe and effective BOSU workouts:

- Working out on BOSU's are safe for the general population, however, it may not be suitable in the case of certain medical conditions. BOSU workouts should then be either modified or avoided.

  Note: Children should be supervised during BOSU training

- Regardless of age and form: Do start with the easiest exercises at first in order to get used to BOSU training and improve the balance before more difficult exercises. This way falls and risky, inefficient workouts are avoided.

- If you feel discomfort or pain during the workout, stop immediately. Change the exercise or stop exercising depending on the nature of the problem.

- Everybody can have a day, when balance and form is at a lower level. Then stick with some easier exercises to avoid getting injured.

- The BOSU dome should be firmly inflated, 8-10 inches high.

- Use the BOSU on a level, clean surface. Carpet, rubber or wood surfaces work best.

- BOSU Fitness, LCC, recommends working out on the dome side and avoid working out standing on the platform side due to the risk of falls and injuries.

- There should be enough, plenty, of space around the BOSU. There should be room for the entire body, arms and legs to move freely in any direction.

- BOSU workout wear should fit, be comfortable and allow safe and effective movement. Avoid clothing that may slip during seated or lying positions on the dome.

- Train in bare feet, during core training and stretching, or use indoor sports shoes or FiveFingers. Wipe off the soles, so there are no pebbles, bits of glass a.o, before putting your feet on the BOSU, to avoid the dome from puncturing. *Note: When you jump (on the floor), shoes may be better. Do not work out in socks or in bare sweaty feet as you may slip and injure yourself.*

- Sweat will make the BOSU slippery, so wipe off sweat from the BOSU (and the floor) during the workout. A dry contact surface provides for a safer training.

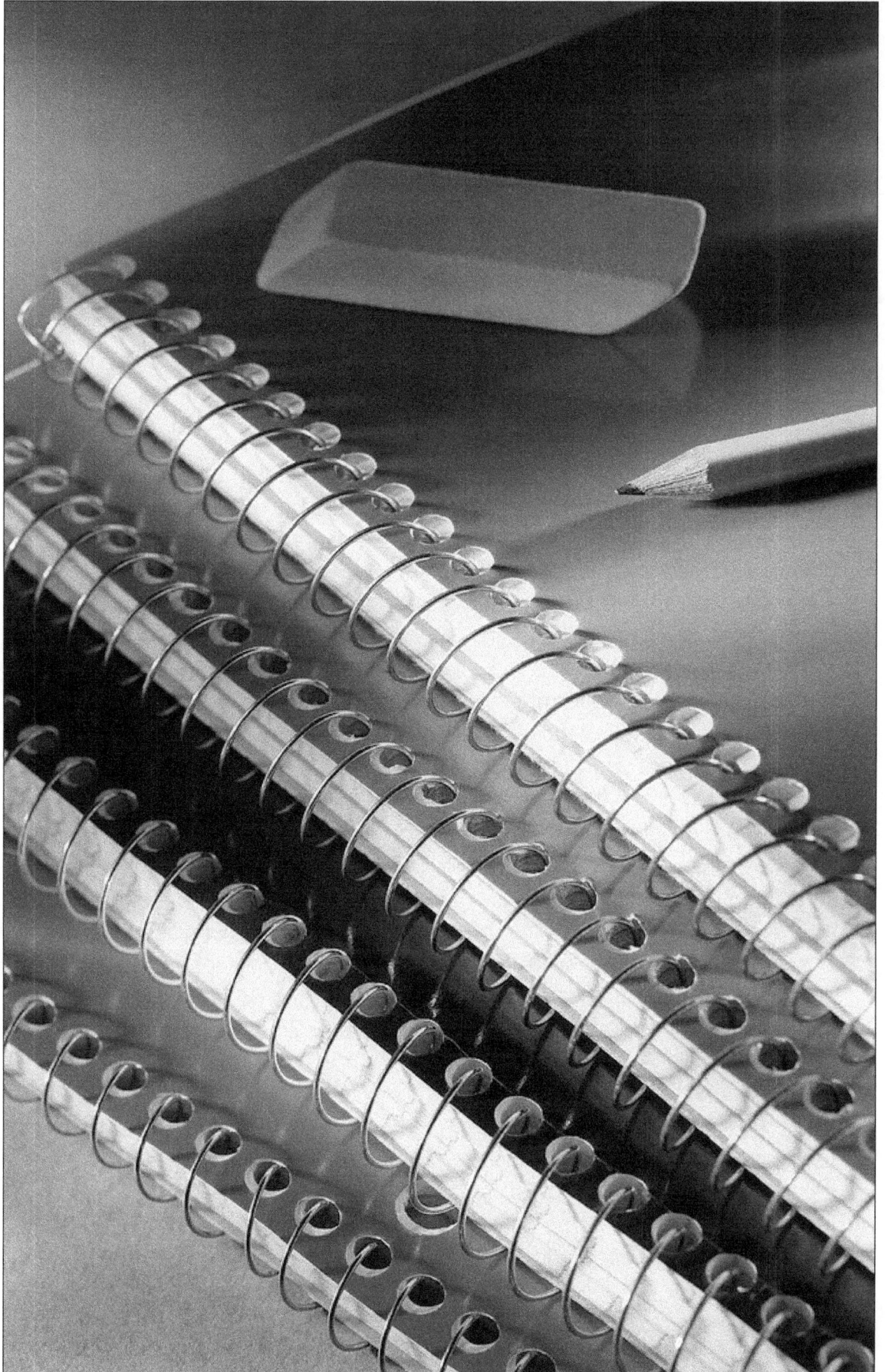

CHAPTER 4 | **PROGRAM DESIGN**

BOSU workouts can be designed in many different ways for fun fitness classes. At the same time classes should be designed with health and sports science principles in mind, always with the health of the exerciser as the top priority.

BOSU workouts for basic training for sports must be planned carefully. Exercises should be chosen with care to fit the athlete and the overall training plan, so the BOSU training complements and improves other training and competitive activities.

Training on an unstable surface is an excellent addition to a fitness program, but should be regarded as such; a supplement to stable surface training. Analyze the demands of the sport and plan accordingly.

For BOSU general fitness workouts there are no strict requirements in regard to format and content, but the exercises should still be selected carefully with the goal and target group in mind, though.

In group fitness the exercises should be demonstrated at more levels; at the easiest level for new exercisers.

MUSIC

BOSU workouts formats:
1) one-on-one-, personal, training, without music,
2) one-on-one or small groups in the gym with 'background music' and
3) group exercise with music
(or sometimes without music).

BOSU workouts can include cardio, strength, stability and flexibility training, therefore the music, too, can range from pop, rock, disco and techno to new age music.

The music, genre, tempo and even volume should be adapted for the exercises, so it enhances workout performance and motivation.
As a general guideline use a moderate tempo, around 120-130 BPM, beats per minute. Play music at a moderate or low volume, especially during exercise cues.

Music can improve motivation. However, it can also be an advantage to exercise without music, as silence is relaxing – a nice break from too much noise during the everyday – and it may make it easier to 'listen to the body' and work out at ones own pace, not that of the music.

PROGRAM VARIABLES

Program design factors for one-on-one as well as group exercise:

- Exercises
- Repetitions
- Sets
- Tempo
- Rest-pauses

Each factor can be varied in many different ways according to the workout goal.

The workouts can focus on strength or strength-endurance, cardio or a combination. And the format can be either continuus or interval training.

EXERCISES

Select the exercises according to the goal and the target group.

In group exercise the instructor should demo each exercise at three levels, easy, intermediate and difficult (hard), *differentiated teaching,* so each participant work out at a suitable level.

The load can be changed from light or moderate to heavy by changing the external load or the lever.

A typical number of exercises is 6-10. When the exercises are simple and not too intense, you can include from 8-16 different exercises.

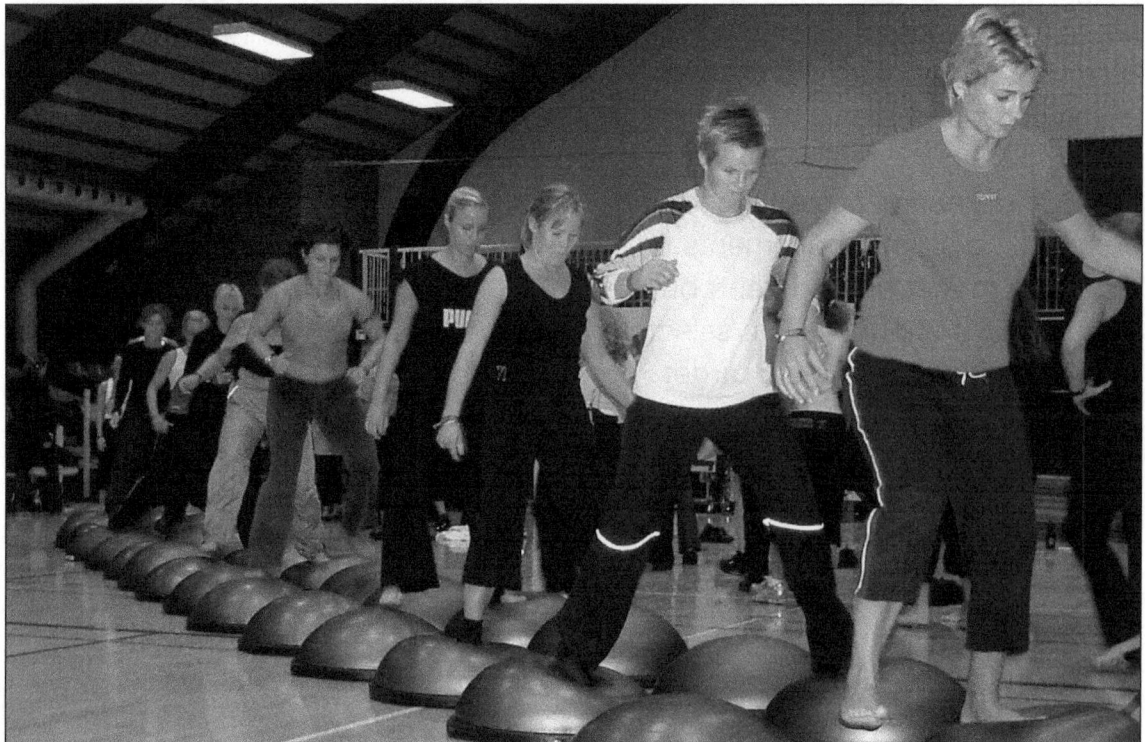

REPETITIONS

A repetition is one full cycle of the exercise from start to finish. The number of *repetitions* determines the workout result:

1-8 repetitions: Strength

12-20+ repetitions: Endurance

8-12 repetitions: General fitness

BOSU strength workouts are quite intense and involve more muscles than strength training in machines, so the recommended number of repetitions is from 6-12. Depending on form and exercise goal, you can perform either fewer or more repetitions than that.

To progress initially you increase the number of repetitions, but when you reach a certain number, increase the load or difficulty instead.

Note: The trainer can recommend a number of repetitions and should also point out, that the exerciser should stop, as soon as he or she feels unable to continue with proper form and correct exercise technique.

SET

A set is a group of repetitions. The norm is 1-3 sets. Depending on the exercise selection, you could choose to perform 3 sets of one exercise and only 1 set of another.

TEMPO

Exercise tempo affects the intensity as well as the difficulty.
In the beginning you should work out at a moderate tempo in order to be able to control the movement.

For strength exercises the tempo is: 2 seconds concentrically, the muscle shortens, and 2-4 seconds eccentrically, the muscle lengthens.

Note: A slower tempo on top of the BOSU in many instances makes the exercise more difficult.

REST-PAUSES

In order to keep the intensity and not fatique the muscles and nervous system excessively, you rest in between the sets.
The rest-pause norm in general exercise is ½-2 minutes.

Rest-pause options:

1. Stop completely and rest.

2. Walk or do short stretches (2 sec.).

3. Train another muscle group during the pause, staggered training, so you stay active, but work other muscles.

For some advanced strength and balance exercises on the BOSU, with many muscles active, you may need a longer rest-pause.

PROGRESSION

For the optimal workout experience and effect you should plan for a **gradual exercise progression**.

In a training program, initially you start at the easiest level, which for some exercisers mean exercises on the floor, off the BOSU.
Then gradually the load or level of difficulty should be increased from time to time.

In the workout, right after the warm-up, start with the more complex or heavy exercises for the major muscles. Then easier exercises for smaller muscles. And specific 'core training' at the end of the workout.

To many exercisers, even those used to resistance training, BOSU training will be challenging initially, so a cautious start is recommended.

For novices, absolute beginners, an entire series or class with the BOSU may be too hard.
It is recommended that the trainer or instructor 1) shows modifications (on the floor), 2) uses (more) pauses or 3) leads shorter workouts.

When you reach a certain level, you can continue to challenge yourself by performing increasingly difficult exercises – if you want to keep on progressing.
Maintenance is another workout goal and may be the preferred choice of some exercisers.

In general you can make the BOSU exercises harder by changing the body position, making the lever longer and the exercise harder, or you can add external load in the form of barbells, dumbbells, elastic bands or partner resistance.

You can also make the exercises more difficult by gradually reducing the base or points of support, by moving the center of gravity, turning the head or closing the eyes.

If you want to make the workouts more intense, this can be done by increasing either the load or the level of difficulty.
Normally you do not increase both at the same time, even if this is an option in workouts for skilled and fit participants.

You regress an exercise by making it easier. However, it is better to start at an easy level and then progress. In this way you avoid failing, maybe even hurting yourself, and having to 'step down' to an easier exercise.

VARIABLES

For variety and increased challenge:

- increase the balance challenge by one or more factors
- increase the difficulty, level of coordination
- increase the number of repetitions
- increase the load
- increase or decrease the tempo

BOSU Balance Challenge Variables
(adapted from BOSU, 2006):

Contact points

- First stabilize with the arms or the legs on the floor.

- First more, then fewer contact points; with both arms and legs, then with one arm or one leg at a time.
  Maybe a BodyBar for support.

- First with support, then unsupported: Hands or feet on the BOSU or floor, then lifted.

Visual affect

- First with open eyes, then with closed eyes.
  Or close one eye at a time.

- First facing forward, focusing on a fixed point, then turning the head or the torso.

Movement

- Body and limbs close to the BOSU, short lever, then longer.

- First the legs, or the arms, then add arm (leg) movements – and torso movements.

- First sagittal, forward-backward, then diagonal and transversal movements.

- First simple, isolated exercises, then complex exercises and sports movements.

External stimulus

- Add external load, use balls, use balls for support, a.o.

- Partner resistance or partner assistance.

VARIATIONS

Exercises can be varied in several ways during the warm-up, cardio, strength, balance, strength and/or flexibility sections of the workout:

- Tempo
- Rhythm
- Direction
- Travelling
- Planes
- Balance
- Joint movement
- Number of active muscles

TEMPO

The tempo may be slow, moderate or fast. Initially the workout tempo should be moderate, not too fast or too slow. Adapt the tempo to the goal and the target group. If it is too fast, it is difficult to perform the exercise with control, if it is too slow, it is hard to keep the balance. *Note: Exercise tempo is not always the same as the music tempo.*

RHYTHM

The exercises can be performed in various tempos and rhythms. E.g. the concentric and eccentric phase in a 2:4 or 1:3 beats/seconds tempo – instead of a 1:1 or 2:2 tempo.

DIRECTION

Direction refers to the position of the body in the room; the way you are facing.
Direction changes add variety and challenge coordination.

Example: Stand on the BOSU. Jump. With every jump or a number of jumps, turn, so you are doing a full turn in e.g. 2-16 jumps.

During cardio or resistance work challenge yourself by changing the direction; initially change direction slowly, but as soon as you (or the participants) are able to, change direction more quickly.

TRAVELLING

Travelling can be **vertical**, up and down, or **horizontal**, floor patterns forward, backward, to the side, diagonally and in circles, e.g. walking around the BOSU.

During the warm-up and cardio workouts – and agility work – you can include horizontal travelling across the floor to increase intensity. Travelling can be with or without simultaneous directional changes.

During cardio and resistance training you can include vertical work, e.g. jumps and hops or squats and lunges.

PLANES

The arms, legs and torso can move in different movement planes:

Sagittal   Forward/backward
Frontal   Sidewards
Transversal Horizontal (rotation)

Functional training is based on compound movements and movement planes, not just isolated muscle work.

BALANCE

In BOSU-workouts the balance is trained via changes in the base of support, position of the body, limbs and head, etc.
Extra balance work on the floor, with or without equipment, is an option.

JOINT MOVEMENTS

A balanced workout includes all possible joint movements:

- Flexion
- Extension
- Abduction
- Adduction
- Rotation
- Circumduction

Note: Rotation requires a moderate tempo (initially) to keep muscular control to avoid twists and falls.

NUMBER OF ACTIVE MUSCLES

Exercises can be complex, involving many active muscles, or isolations, few active muscles. And you can use one arm or one leg or both at the same time or alternating.

Bilateral training with both arms or legs working at the same time is time efficient and allows for more exercises in the workout. And you know, that both sides are being trained equally!
However, the disadvantage is, that a strong, dominating side does the majority of the work. Therefore it is also a good idea to do:

Unilateral training, first with one side (arm or leg), then the opposite side. This allows for concentrated, isolated training and stability work.

Note: During unilateral exercises, remember to take an equal number of repetitions for the right and the left side for a balanced workout.

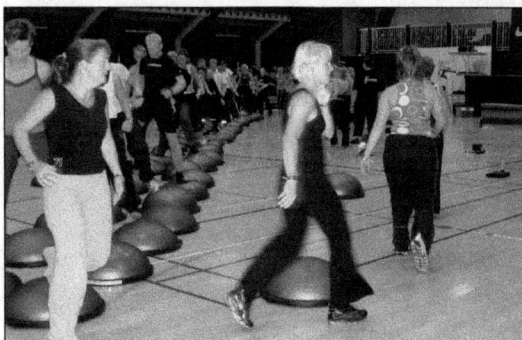

ORGANISATION

Organisation refers to:

1. **Position(ing)** of exerciser(s) and equipment and of exercisers in relation to each other (formation).

   – Individually
   – Pairs
   – Groups, small
   – Team(s), 1-4 big groups

2. **Sequencing**, the order of the exercises and their linking.

3. **Integration** of mats and other equipment.

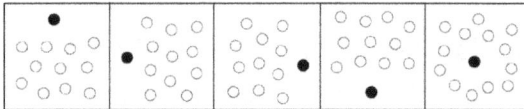

Figure 4.1: Instructor and participant positions.

POSITIONING

In group exercise, the instructor typically is in the front with all the participants facing front, facing the instructor. To add variety and improve learning, it is smart to change position from time to time:
By the front wall, back wall, side walls or in the middle of the room.
It creates the impression of a 'new' class; the participants see the room and each other from a new angle.

Alternate between different positions; in unison and pair, group and team work.
Do not change positions all the time, but do a number of exercises in each position or formation, so you do not have to rush from position to position: Avoid workout stress.

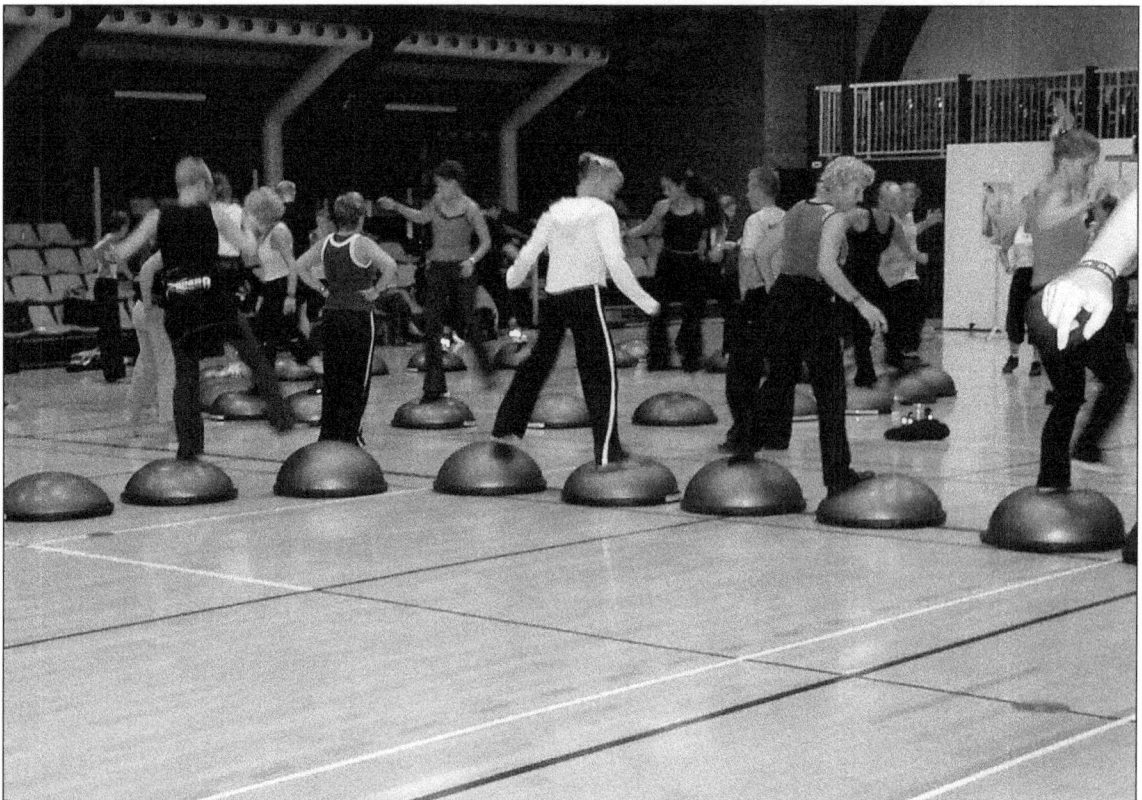

Instructor and participant position:

- In unison (traditional format)
- In line(s)
- In a circle formation
- In pairs or ◯ ◯ ◯ small groups ◯ ◯

In toning and balance workouts, when you are stationary, on the spot, you can use a circle format; this works well, because the instructor is closer to all the participants and easier to see and hear.

The circle format facilitates 'social workouts', the participants can see each other, have eye contact. One disadvantage of circle formats is that they do not work well with travelling patterns.

Partner training

Training with a partner has many advantages. Apart from the social aspect of working together, or competing, you can add extra load, e.g. by having the partner push against you or by lifting the partner.

Note: Some exercisers find it difficult or unpleasant to hold or touch a(nother) sweaty body and hence dislike partner exercises.

Partner exercises can be performed standing (sitting) on a BOSU each doing pushing or pulling exercises. For coordination and balance work exercisers can mirror each other. Or one partner can be on a BOSU, while the other assists, resists or throws balls to the first partner.

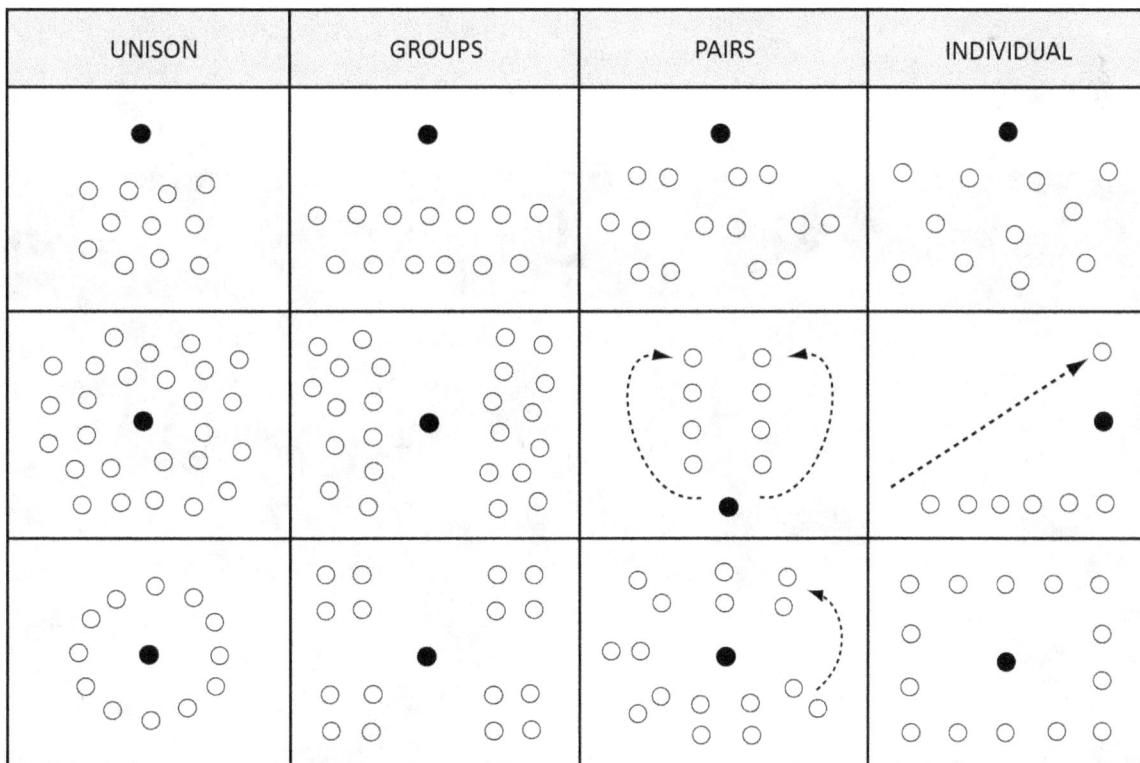

UNISON	GROUPS	PAIRS	INDIVIDUAL

Figure 4.2: Variations; different positions and travelling patterns.

Starting positions

BOSU exercises can be performed from different starting positions; different starting positions adds variety to the BOSU-program. Choose starting position according to the exercise and choose the positions with maximal effect – avoid ineffective exercises.

The exercises can be sequenced, so they start from the same starting position in order to have as few changes as possible; avoid rushing from one position to another, up and down, with too many position changes within a limited time period.

Create a structured harmonious workout, which is motivating and easy to follow.

- Standing (on floor) facing front (behind BOSU, face forward)
- Standing beside the BOSU
- Standing in front of the BOSU
- Standing, feet staggered; one on the floor, one on the BOSU
- Standing on the BOSU
- Half kneeling on the BOSU
- All fours on the BOSU
- Kneeling on the BOSU
- Sitting on the BOSU
- Supine on the BOSU
- Side-lying on the BOSU
- Prone on the BOSU

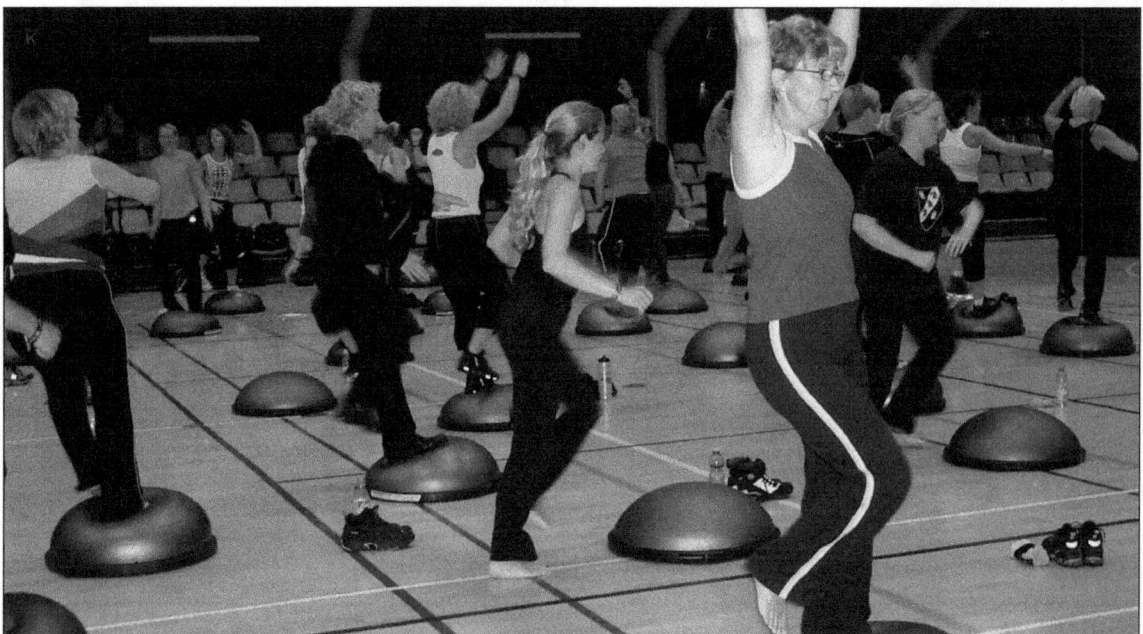

SEQUENCING

The exercises should be sequenced, in a logical order in respect to the muscles used (complexity and load) and body position.
Avoid changing position too many times. This seems unorganized and can be difficult to follow for novices. Exception: Advanced circuit type classes.

In cardio and agility workouts with lots of travelling forward and back-ward, to the side and diagonally, the exercisers should be able move in unison and everybody should be able to see the instructor.

INTEGRATION

BOSU workouts may include other equipment.
Free weights and elastic resistance provides more options for strength training, while balls, therapy boards, wobble boards etc. increases the level of difficulty and the number of stability work options.

The equipment can be used in the BOSU exercises or in between, or after, on the floor without the BOSU. Using equipment while on the BOSU requires some proficiency and a good balance; the exercisers should be able to control the movements.

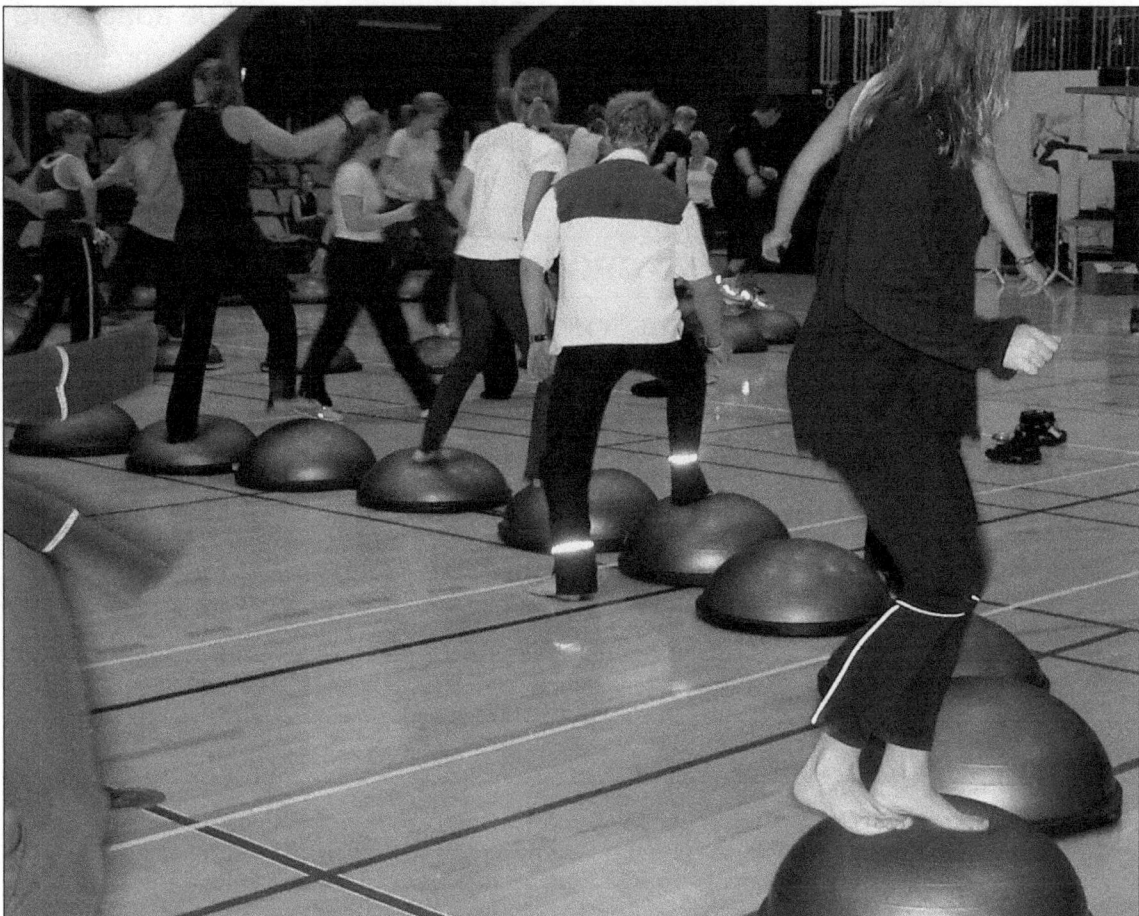

CHAPTER 5 | CLASS DESIGN

BOSU work can be included in group exercise classes, e.g. body toning or circuit classes, or you can design an all BOSU workout.

The structure of an all BOSU class may vary; below is an example of an all-round fitness BOSU class (see Appendix):

5-15   minute warm-up
20-30 minute cardio
10-20 minute resistance and
         balance work
5-10   minute cool-down/stretch

The warm-up may be of shorter or longer duration depending on the workout and the participants.

Cardio work should be followed by a cool-down (I), easy movements, which gradually lowers the heart rate to resting level.

Resistance training can be with or without the BOSU and with or without additional equipment.

Balance and stability is trained during cardio and resistance work, so additional balance work is not necessary.

Stretching – and relaxation – adds a nice wellness conclusion to a class. The stretches should be adapted to the class goals and the exercisers. Stretching serves as a relaxing and pleasurable cooldown (II).

BOSU ALL-ROUND GROUP EXERCISE PROGRAM		
PHASE	**DURATION**	**MUSIC TEMPO**
Introduction	1-2 minutes	No music
Warm-up	7-15 minutes	120-130 BPM
Cardio (cool-down I)	20+ minutes	120-135 BPM
Resistance training	10-20+ minutes	90-130 BPM
Balance work	0-15 minutes	90-130 BPM
Cooldown (II)/Stretch	3-15+ minutes	< 110 BPM
Outro	1-2 minutes	No music

Table 5.1: BOSU allround class. Class structure example. Cardio exercise should be followed by a cooldown (I), which lowers the heart rate gradually. At the end of class there is a final cooldown (II) with stretching and relaxation. In this example balance work is shown as a separate part of class, but it is (also) an integral part of BOSU cardio and resistance work. Aagaard, 2010.

CHAPTER 6 | WARM-UP

WARM-UP

The workout starts with a warm-up, physical and mental preparation for the activity to follow.

Physically the warm-up raises the heart rate, increases the blood flow, and oxygen supply, to the muscles, and makes the tissues more resilient. This enhances performance and reduces the risk of injury.

Mentally you prepare for the workout and start to focus on the exercises.

General warm-ups include:

- Rhythmic limbering
- Muscle isolations
- Dynamic stretches

Rhythmic limbering involves movement of the large muscles groups, the legs; *low impact* impact moves without running/jumping for the first five minutes for a gradual start.

Muscle isolations include dynamic upper body (and some lower body) movements.

Select appropriate stretches for the activity to come; warm-up stretches should be active and dynamic to raise the heart rate and prepare the muscles and joints for movement.

Specific warm-up involves getting the body prepared for the specific exercises in the workout.

Apart from general exercises you should perform movemens similar to the exercises in the workout, e.g. the same movements with a smaller, gradually increasing range of motion.

The design of the warm-up depends on the workout; is it a high intensity sports workout or more of a traditional stationary workout with basic strength and stability exercises?

In fitness group exercise the general and speciific warm-up is often integrated for an allround warm-up.

In group exercise warm-up moves can be taught using 1) linear progression, you take one thing at a time and do not combine the exercises, or 2) block choreography in which arm, leg and core movements are mixed and combined into little (4 x 8 beats) combinations.

METHOD

Warm-ups should start at the easiest level – specific to the exerciser(s) – and be progressed gradually:

Intensity, a.o. tempo, range of motion and travelling.

Impact on the bones and joints should be 'low impact' for the first part of the warm-up (at least 5 min.). *Note.: Impact is not the same as intensity; the impact on the joints may be low even if the intensity is moderate or high.*

Coordination. Include 'rehearsel moves' for the workout; exercises and parts of exercises at an easier level – provide a feeling of success.

CONTENT

The core muscles are central in BOSU workouts: In BOSU warm-ups you should therefore include:

• Spinal flexion
• Spinal extension
• Lateral flexion
• Rotations

As well as movements for the other major joints.

The exerciser(s) should be warmed up in an easy and meaningful, motivating, way.
The easier you start, the easier it is to progress with success.

The warm-up should avoid:

- Uncontrolled and fast ballistic movements.

- Static stretches, as they make the heart rate drop.

- Isometric strength exercises 'slows down' the warm-up and feels hard and de-motivating.

During the warm-up you should focus on posture and technique.

The instructor and exercisers should be aware of and **avoid these common mistakes:**

- Protruding head

- Elevated shoulders

- Exaggerated spinal flexion or (hyper)extension

- Locking of the joints, e.g. knees and elbows

- Uncontrolled ballistic movement

DURATION

The duration of the warm-up should match the rest of the workout.

The duration of fitness warm-ups should be approximately 15 % of total workout time; for a 60 minute workout this would be 9 minutes.

The general recommendation for group exercise is **7-10 minutes.**

The warm-up may be shorter, around 5-8 minutes, depending on the exercises, intensity and total duration.

The warm-up may be longer, if the instructor or trainer wishes to use the warm-up for technique drills or special exercises.

Especially in BOSU-workouts for weaker or older target groups, the participants may need a longer more gradual warm-up.

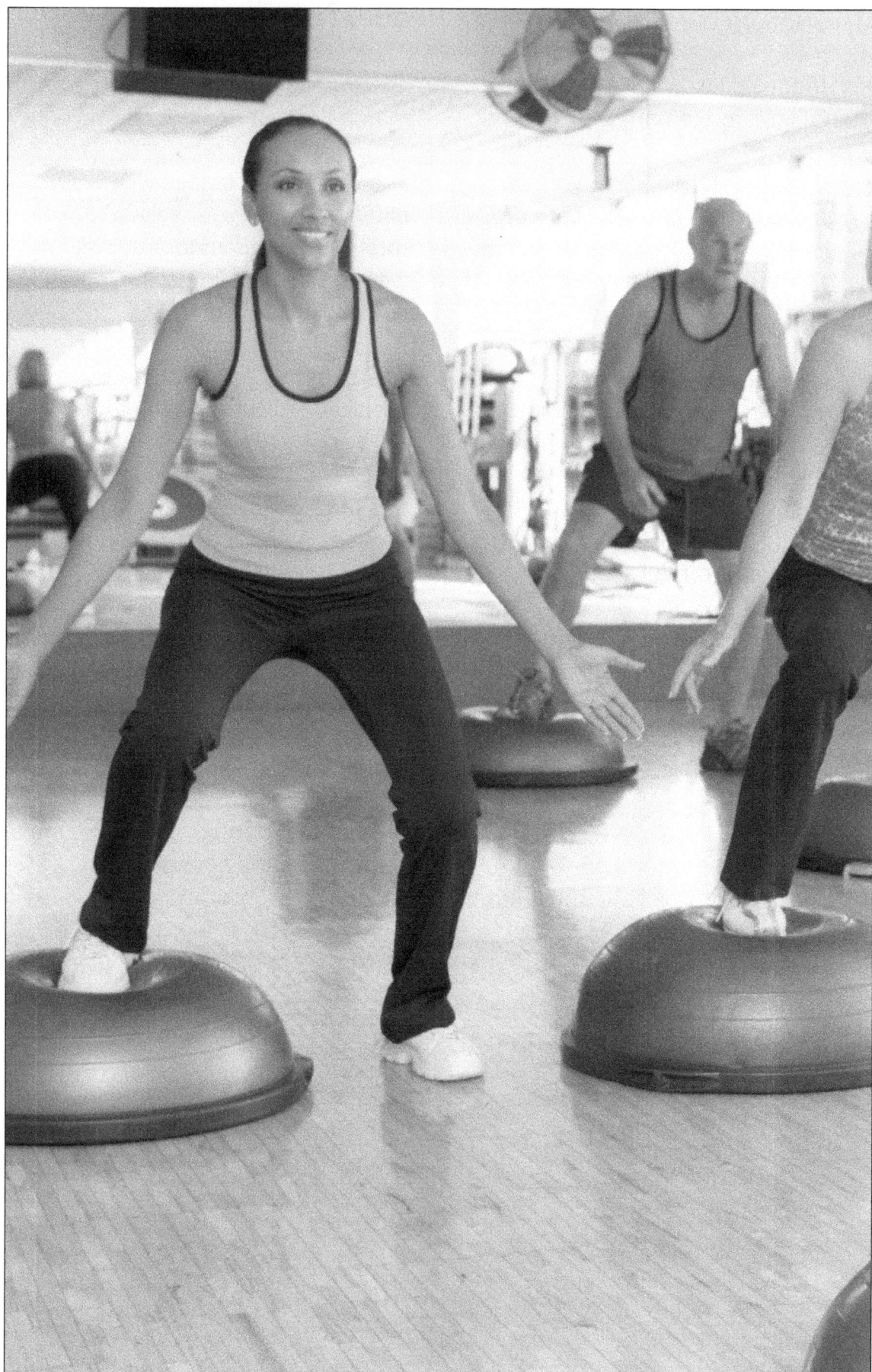

CHAPTER 7 | CARDIO

Cardio workouts with coordination and balance work on the BOSU, for individuals and groups, can look like step training; with step patterns

- up and down from the BOSU
- on top of the BOSU
- over and up and over the BOSU
- around the BOSU

Basic steps are **walking, jogging, hopping and jumping** on the floor and on the top of the BOSU.

You can also include step training movements like *step hamstring curl, kneelift, skip and kick, abduction, extension (hip), step lunge, mambo and over the top.*

All steps can be performed in either **low impact**, without running and jumping or **high impact**, with hops and jumps. Steps and impact should be selected according to the target group and workout goals.

Tips for higher intensity cardio work:

- **Many active muscles**, especially the large muscles of the legs. Combine leg work with upper body movements for a 5-10 % increase in energy consumption.

- **Vertical movement of COG**, the centre of gravity, up (and down) raises the heart rate fast.

- **Hortizontal travelling.** Movements around the BOSU, across the floor, from side to side, forward and backward, diagonally and in patterns.

- **Tempo.** Simple slow movements can increase the heart rate, but a faster movement tempo will raise the heart rate more and faster. *Note: The movement tempo should be adapted to the target group; you should never work so fast, that you lose control and reduce the workload and effect – and risk injury.*

- **Full range of motion,** aim for full range of motion.

DURATION

The duration of the cardio part of a class may vary depending on the intensity, which again depends on the workout goal and target group.

Recommended duration for BOSU cardio work is 20-30 minutes.

Basic step
Walk up and down

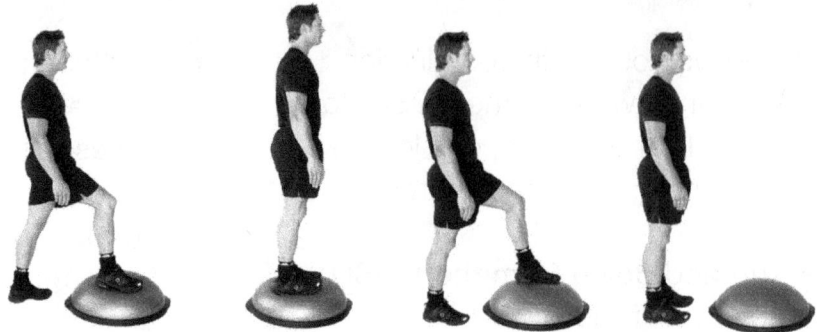

Step curl

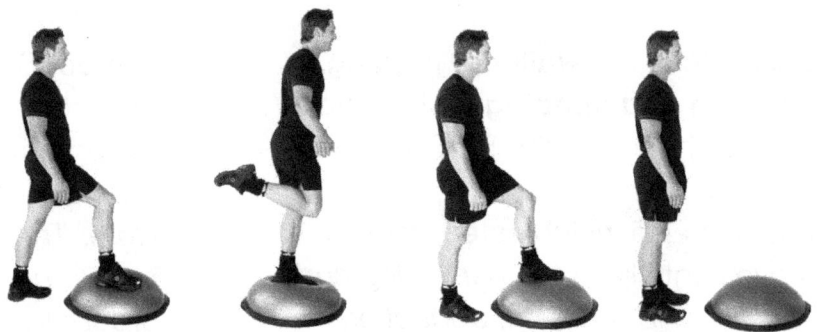

Step skip

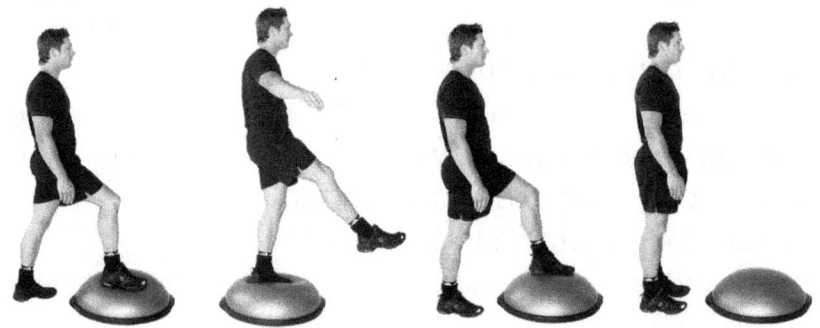

Step kneelift

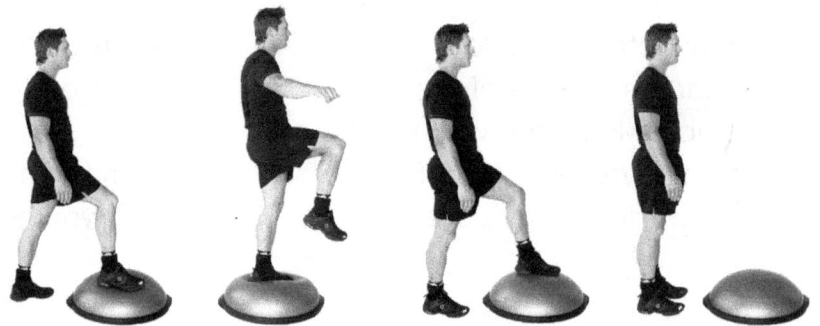

TECHNIQUE	NOTE	VARIATION
Walk up and down the BOSU, BOSU stepping. Same foot leads every time: 1. First foot up. 2. Second foot up. 3. First foot down. 4. Second foot down.	Step up onto a stable position on the top. Keep knees and feet aligned. First step should allow some room for the second foot up; body centered on the BOSU. Step with an erect posture, so it is easier to keep the balance.	Different arm/body exercises. Rhythm. Direction. Travelling (e.g. from BOSU to BOSU).
1. First foot up. 2. Second foot to buttocks; hamstring curl. 3. Second foot down. 4. First foot down. The lead has now been changed; opposite foot is ready to step up.	Step up onto the centre of the BOSU dome. Keep knee and foot aligned. Step with an erect posture, so it is easier to keep the balance.	Different arm/body exercises. Rhythm, repeater; 2, 3, 4, 5, 6, 7 repetitions (curls). A 3-repeater; up, curl/tap to floor/curl/tap/curl, down, down fits the music, an 8-count, perfectly. Direction. Travelling.
1. First foot up. 2. Second foot forward, knee extension; skip. 3. Second foot down. 4. First foot down. The lead has now been changed; opposite foot is ready to step up.	Contract the thigh, extend the knee with control. Step up onto the centre of the BOSU dome. Keep knee and foot aligned. Step with an erect posture, so it is easier to keep the balance.	Different arm/body exercises. Rhythm, repeaters; 2, 3, 4, 5, 6, 7 repetitions (skips). Direction. Travelling.
1. First foot up. 2. Second foot/knee is lifted, kneelift above horizontal. 3. Second foot down. 4. First foot down. The lead has now been changed; opposite foot is ready to step up.	Lift the knee above horizontal for higher intensity. Step up onto the centre of the BOSU dome. Keep knee and foot aligned. Step with an erect posture, so it is easier to keep the balance.	Different arm/body exercises. Rhythm, repeaters; 2, 3, 4, 5, 6, 7 repetitions (kneelifts). Direction. Travelling.

Step kick

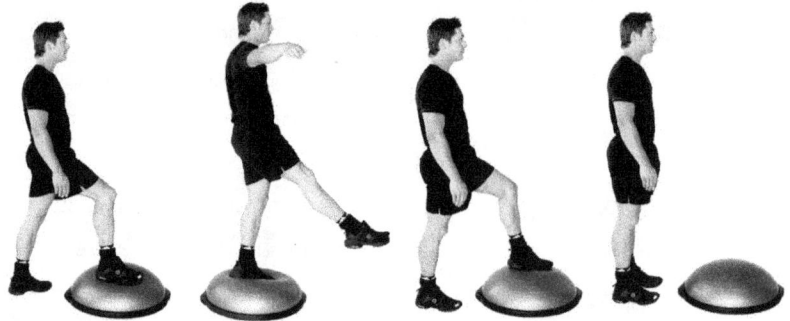

Step extension

Step abduction

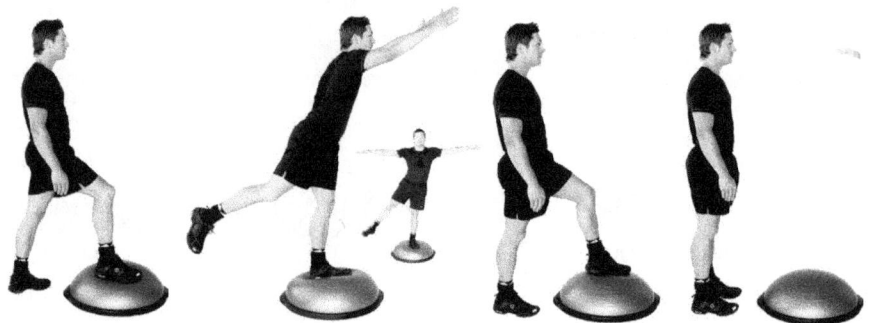

Step out jack

Sidelunge
from the top

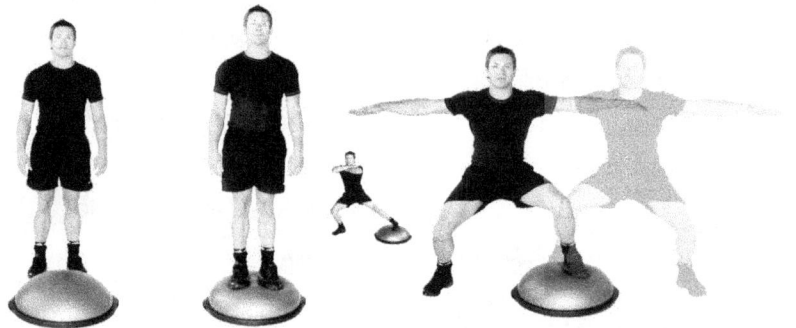

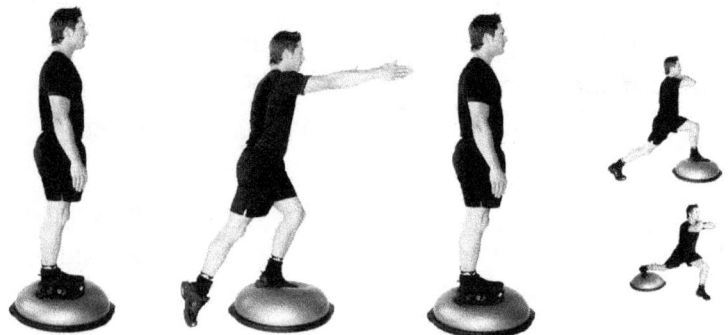

Step lunge
(basic lunge)

Lunge
from the top

TECHNIQUE	NOTE	VARIATION
1. First foot up. 2. Second leg forward, straight leg lift; kick (front). 3. Second foot down. 4. First foot down. The lead has now been changed; opposite foot is ready to step up.	Keep the kicking-leg straight, muscle contracted throughout the exercise; it increases the intensity. Step up onto the centre. Keep knee and foot aligned. Step with a good posture; it is easier to keep the balance.	Different arm/body exercises. Rhythm, repeaters; 2, 3, 4, 5, 6, 7 repetitions (kicks). Direction. Travelling.
1. First foot up. 2. Second leg backward, straight leg hip extension. 3. Second foot down. 4. First foot down. The lead has now been changed; opposite foot is ready to step up.	Hip extension range of motion max. 5-15 degr.; contract the core, do not arch the back. Step up onto the centre. Keep knee and foot aligned. Step with a good posture; it is easier to keep the balance.	Different arm/body exercises. Rhythm, repeaters; 2, 3, 4, 5, 6, 7 repetitions (extensions). Direction. Travelling. **Leg abduction.** Leg out.
Standing on the top. 1. Take a lunge step to the side, to the floor, as a jumping jack; both legs bent. 2. Push off, back to the top. 3. Lunge step opposite leg. 4. Push off, back to the top.	Contract the thigh muscles and keep knees and feet aligned at all times. Avoid twisting the knees. Keep an erect posture.	Different arm/body exercises. Rhythm. Direction. Travelling. **Rock step (push step)** Stand beside the BOSU. Step up, push off forcefully, lift foot or step down, e.g. all the way around the BOSU. Repeat with the opposite leg.
1. First foot up. 2. Second foot up. 3. First foot lunge back. 4. First foot return to the top. 5. Second foot lunge back. 6. Second foot return. 7. First foot steps down. 8. Second foot steps down.	Tap only; touch the toes lightly to the floor; do not step down; avoid overstretching the achilles tendon.	Different arm/body exercises. Rhythm, repeaters (2, 3, 4, 5, 6, 7 repetitions (kick). Direction. Strength lunges from the floor to the BOSU, or from the top to the floor. *Note: Avoid/limit forward lunges from the top as this is hard on the knees.*

Walk
on the top

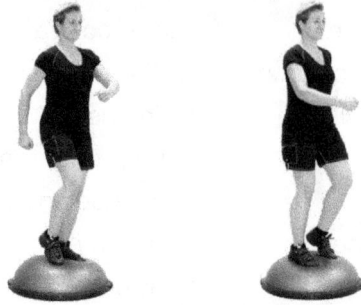

Jog
on the top

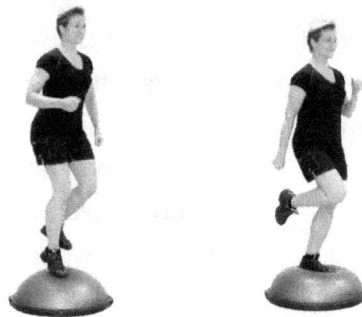

Hopscotch
on the top

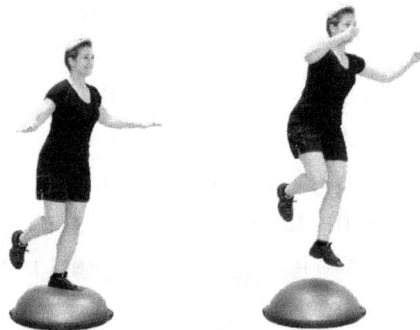

Jump
on the top

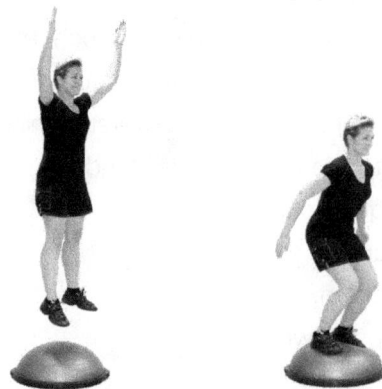

TECHNIQUE	NOTE	VARIATION
Walk on the top. Distribute the weight evenly across the feet. Keep the torso upright. Stabilize. Move the arms dynamically.	Keep knees and feet aligned. Avoid twisting the knees.	Different arm/body exercises. Tempo. Rhythm. Direction. Travelling.
Jog on the top. Distribute the weight evenly across the feet. Keep the torso upright. Stabilize. Move the arms dynamically.	Keep knees and feet aligned. Avoid twisting the knees.	Different arm/body exercises. Tempo. Rhythm. Direction. Travelling.
Standing on one leg at the top. The foot is centrered on the top. Hop on one foot; hop two or more times on each foot, then change. Keep the upper body erect. Contract the core, stabilize. Move the arms dynamically.	Hop 2, 3, 4 on each foot; not too many in a row; avoid fatigue and falls. Keep knees and feet aligned. Avoid twisting the knees.	Different arm/body exercises. Tempo. Rhythm. Direction. Travelling.
Standing on the top. Feet slightly apart. Jump; bend and extend the legs quickly and jump. Land with soft knees. Keep the torso erect. Contract the core, stabilize. Use the arms to increase jump height and for balance.	Keep the torso erect; this makes jumping easier. Land with soft/bent knees. Keep knees and feet aligned. Avoid twisting the knees. Contract the pelvic floor during the jumps (landings).	**Jump (hop) turn** Jump up and turn 1/8, 1/4 or 1/2 (1/1) and land on the BOSU. Repeat one or more times. Repeat the opposite way. **Freestyle jumps on the top** E.g. jump as high as possible (as you can safely jump).

EXERCISE

Twist
on the top

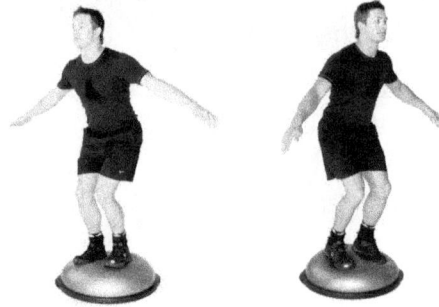

Jump up
from floor to top

Jump over (forward)

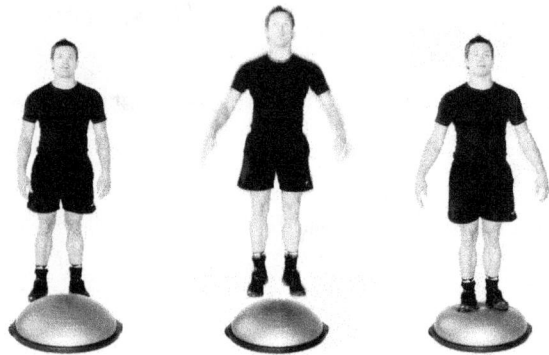

Over the top

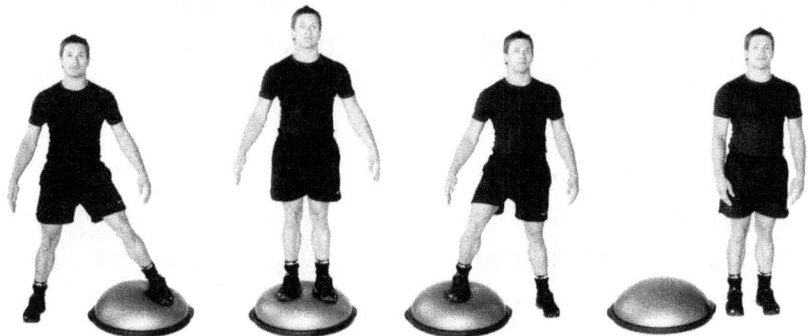

Jump over the top
(lateral movement)

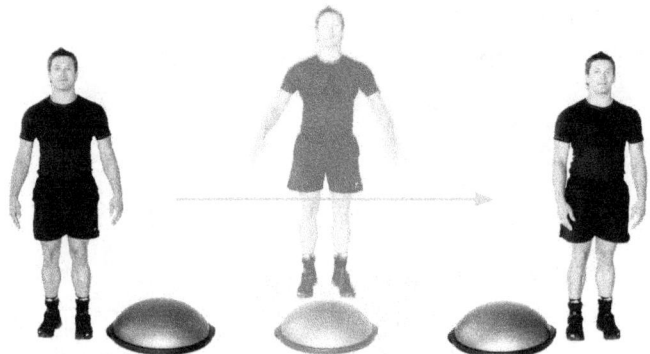

TECHNIQUE	NOTE	VARIATION
Standing on the top. Feet hip-width apart and centered at the top. Jump and at the same time twist from side to side. Land with legs slightly bent. Keep the torso erect. Use the arms for balance.	Maintain good posture; it is easier to jump and twist. Twist with control, knees and feet aligned. Avoid twisting the knees. Contract the pelvic floor when jumping hard and repeatedly.	Different arm/body exercises. Tempo. Rhythm. Direction.
Standing behing the BOSU. Bend/extend the legs quickly and jump onto the BOSU. Land with legs slightly bent. Keep the torso erect. Contract the core, stabilize. Use the arms – for jumping higher and keeping balance.	Maintain good posture; it is easier to jump. Twist with control, knees and feet aligned. Avoid twisting the knees. Contract the pelvic floor when jumping hard and repeatedly.	Different arm/body exercises. Tempo. Rhythm. Direction. Travelling (e.g. over more BOSU's) Variation: Hop over BOSU, ½ hop turn. Repeat, return.
Standing beside the BOSU. Step laterally onto the BOSU; first foot up makes room for the second foot. Step down at the opposite side. Contract the core, stabilize. Use the arms for jumping higher and keeping balance.	Can be performed in low impact, without jogging and jumping, or high impact. On the last, fourth step, the leg can be lifted (knee, heel etc.). Move with control. Keep knees and feet aligned at all times. Avoid twisting the knees.	Different arm movements. Tempo, direction. **Squat push-away** Standing beside the BOSU. Lunge-squat up with one foot. Push forcefully back. Repeat. After a set repeat with the opposite leg.
Standing beside the BOSU. Bend/extend the legs quickly and jump over the BOSU. Land with soft knees. Torso erect. Contract the core and the pelvic floor, when jumping hard and repeatedly. Use the arms for power.	Progression: 1. Step over the BOSU, low. 2. Jog laterally over BOSU. 3. Jump over the BOSU and pause before jumping back. 4. Jump side to side without pausing. Controlled jumping. Keep knees and feet aligned.	**Squat ½ hop** Standing, sumo position, one foot up, one foot down. Hop up, turn ½, land in the same spot, but facing the other way. Repeat.

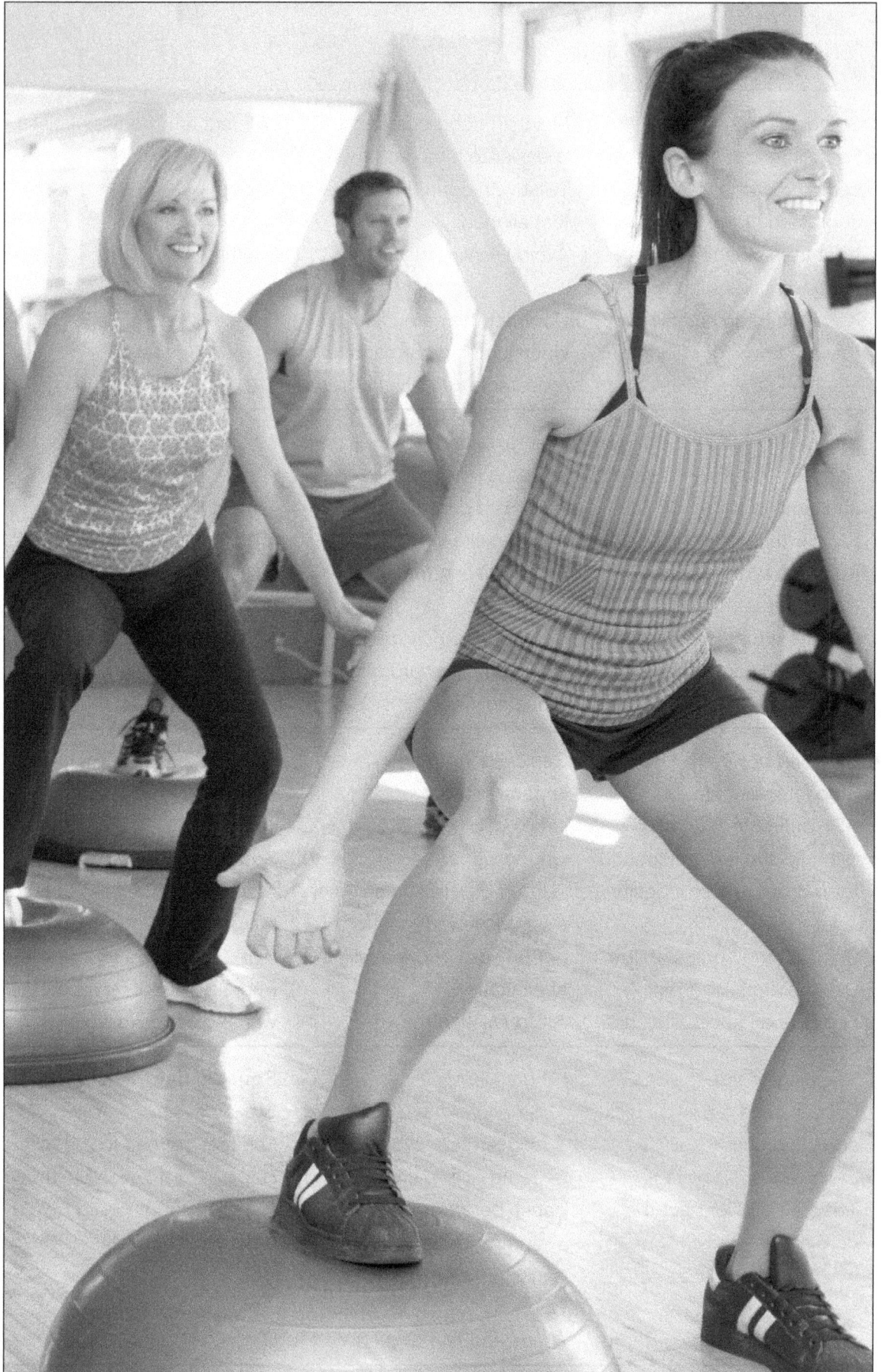

CHAPTER 8 | **COORDINATION**

COORDINATION TRAINING

Coordination training includes arm-and-leg coordination, muscular control, precision and timing, rhythm, spacial awareness and balance.

During BOSU-workouts it is possible to train all of these areas, however, typically the workout focuses on balance and stability work.

Coordination training is integrated in most exercises of the warm-up, cardio, strength, stability and core work and in some instances in the cool-down and stretching exercises.

BALANCE TRAINING

BOSU-training *is* balance training. During all exercises on the BOSU, your senses and muscles are working to stabilize the body.
Balance training can be dynamic, with movement, or static, without movement (of supporting bodypart).

During the warm-up you can do easy dynamic balance work on the floor, with or without the BOSU.

Tip: Select easy warm-up exercises for a motivating start for beginners and advanced exercisers alike.

At beginning level you can perform walking steps, steps up and down the BOSU in a moderate tempo. They can be coupled with short standing 'balances' on the top with feet shoulder-width apart.

At intermediate level you can stand on one or both legs on the top and keep the balance, while moving the arms or the torso – with the eyes open or closed.

At advanced level it is possible to perform jogs, hops and jumps on and off the BOSU, a.o. 'jump and stick' exercises and hops and jumps with turns.

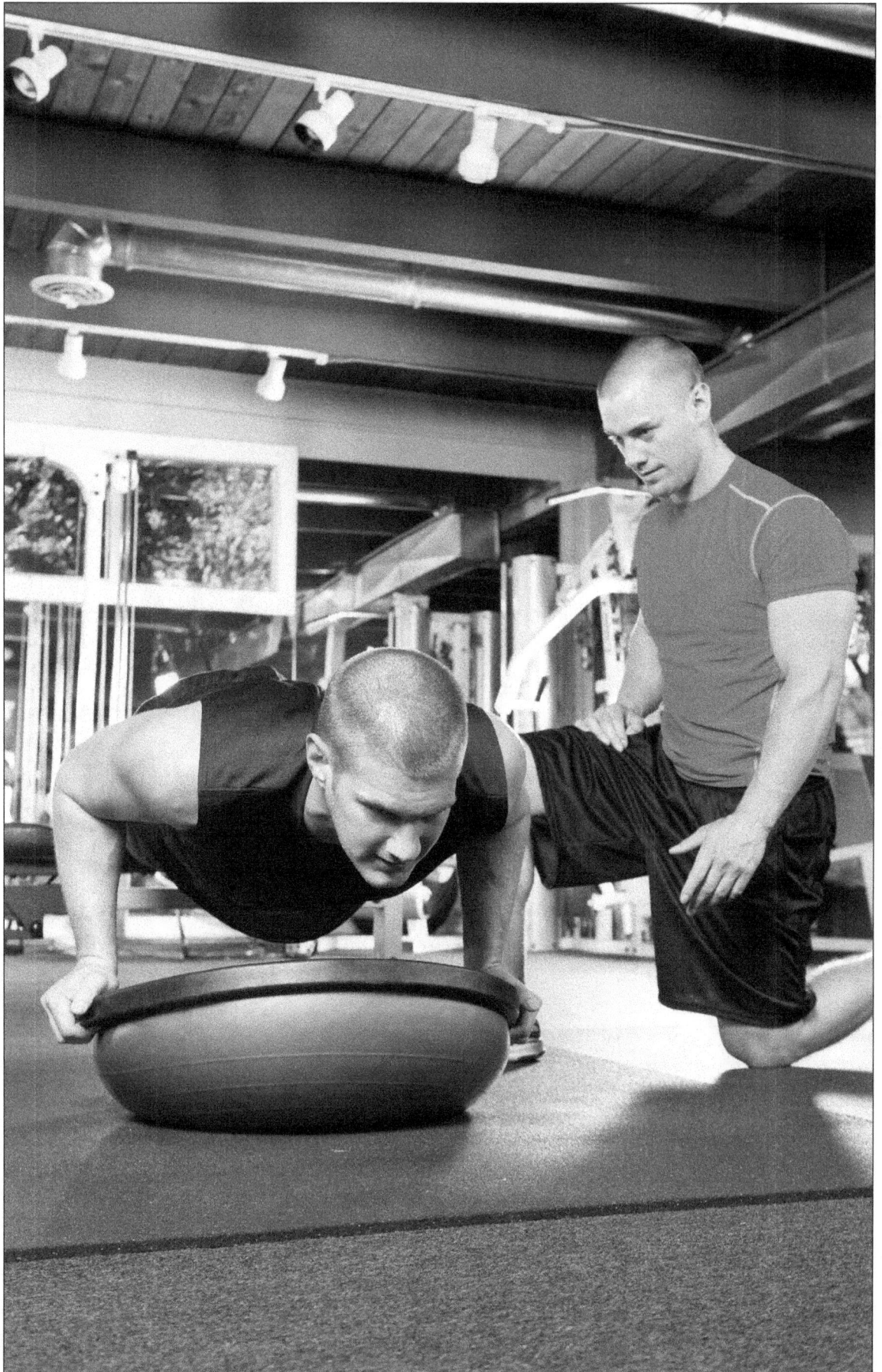

CHAPTER 9 | **STRENGTH**

STRENGTH TRAINING

BOSU training can be designed as an all strength training workout, for individuals or group. Or you can use the BOSU for strength or core training during the resistance training section, 5-15 minutes, of other workouts; aerobics, step training, fitness boxing, circuit training, a.o.

Strength training on the BOSU is challenging, so you need a certain level of fitness and preparation.

Program design. Select:

1. A number of exercises specific to the time available and goal and target group.

2. The right exercises for the goal and target group.

3. Less demanding exercises, if scheduled after other heavy or intense training.

4. Relatively few repetitions, 6-12, and sets, 1-3.
   30-90 seconds rest-pause between sets depending on the exercise and the intensity.

5. A functional and safe sequence.

6. A moderat tempo, not too fast or too slow initially. Correct exercise technique should be maintained.

EXERCISE SELECTION

A major advantage of strength training with the BOSU is, that even if you perform traditional exercises for the outer unit muscles, e.g. ab curl, oblique curl and back extension, at the same time you are working the inner unit stabilizers, which contract when you have to keep the balance.

Exercises:

Isometric exercises, planks in many positions, which are held for longer or shorter periods of time. One or more repetitions.

Dynamic exercises with muscle shortening and lengthening; concentric and eccentric work. Dynamic exercises can be:

Complex exercises for several muscles at a time.

Isolation exercises for one muscle group at a time. This is preferable 1) initially when learning an exercise (part-to-whole principle) and 2) when you want to strengthen a specific area.

Often workouts have both dynamic and isometric (core) exercises; exercises with or without the BOSU, exercises on or off the BOSU and exercises with bodyweight, weights, bands or tubing.

Strength and/or stability: When lifting weights on the BOSU, you will find that you cannot lift as much weight as when on the floor; you are using energy to stabilize yourself on the top. For extra strength training include floor exercises.

A balanced workout: In a workout you should, as a general rule, train 'muscle pairs'; agonists and antagonists, e.g. chest and upper back, abdominals and lower back, biceps and triceps, quads and hamstrings (exception: split programs).
Focus on the muscles with extra need for strengthening; upper back, posterior deltoids, triceps, glutes, hamstrings and abdominals and back extensors.

Exercise sequence: Heavy or more challenging exercises in the beginning, before the neuromuscular system becomes too fatiqued. Then easier exercises.
Specific core training should be performed towards the end of the workout.

EXERCISE TECHNIQUE

For a better workout, better results; start the exercises in the correct starting position (when standing; with an erect posture) with neck and spine in neutral alignment.

Irrespective of your body position; standing, sitting, kneeling or lying, in general – **do not**:

- Stick your head forward, or tilt it forward or backward (unless it is a neck exercise).

- Keep your shoulders raised.

- Let your shoulder blades to glide too much outward or forward.

- Hunch or sway your back excessively or uncontrolled.

- Hyperextend, 'lock' your joints, e.g. knees and elbows.

- Force the joints into faulty or twisted positions.

Recommended exercise tempo in strength training for beginners is: 2-4 seconds for the concentric phase, the muscle is shortening, and 2-4 seconds for the eccentric phase, the muscle is lengthening.

Tip: Over time progress to a faster concentric tempo, e.g. 1 second or explosive.

Movements at a slow to moderate tempo makes it easier for beginners to contract and control the movements, so the exercises work.

Tip: When using music for strength workouts, choose slower music (e.g. 80-120 BPM) and generally perform exercises 'a tempo' with the music or slower – with control.

Typical exercise breathing pattern: Exhale on the work, the concentric phase, inhale on the preparation, or negative work, the eccentric phase. Breathe naturally and keep breathing, also during isometric exercises, do *not* hold your breath.

DURATION

The BOSU workout duration depends on the intensity, the exercises and the structure; is the workout focusing on just one physical aspect, e.g. strength, or is it a hybrid workout, e.g. plus cardio.

BOSU group exercise workout total duration is approx. 50-55 minutes.

The duration of the strength training section can be from 5-35 minutes depending on the workout focus and exercise selection.

Express workouts of 30 minute duration are also an option.

The next six pages list popular BOSU strength exercises. (more in chapter 14, page 81).

The exercises can be performed with or without resistance and be used for one-on-one as well as group exercise.

LOWER BODY EXERCISES

- **Stationary lunge,**
  one foot up, one down

- **Bulgarian squat**
  (back foot on BOSU behind you)

- **Lunge** (step up with one foot)

- **Lunge with kneelift**

- **Lunge forward/backward**
  (up onto top, backward on floor)

- **Lunge back** (from top)
  (reverse lunge)

- **Lunge back** (from top)
  with hip rotation return

- **Lunge back** (from top)
  w/mini-deadlift end-phase

- **Lunge back with kneelift**
  (on top)

- **Side lunge** (from floor)
  (side squat push-away)

- **Side lunge** (from top)
  (sidelunge down and up)

- **Squat on top** (dome squat)

- **Squat with rotation** (on top)

- **Squat hop over squat**
  (squat across)

- **Squat hop-turn squat**
  (squat flip switch)

- **Squat jump with hold** (stick)

LOWER BODY EXERCISES

- Jump twist
  (skiing moguls)

- Jump with turn, floor
  onto top (1/8, 1/4, ½)

- Jump on top with
  turning (1/8, 1/4, ½)

- Jump/hop freestyle

- Rock step from front
  (one foot up, one down, 'rock')

- Rock step from side
  (push into the BOSU)

- Rock step 'around the world'

- Standing hip-abduction

- Sidelying hip-abduction

- Squat to hip-abduction
  (bend, extend and sidelift)

- Three-point
  hip-extension

- Prone
  hip-extension

- Prone (extension)
  hand-to-foot touch

- Dynamic bridge
  (BOSU up or down)

- Static, isometric, bridge
  (BOSU up or down)

- Bridge with 'rocking'
  (tilt the BOSU form side to side)

- Bridge with circle
  (BOSU on the dome side)

UPPER BODY EXERCISES

- Standing shoulderpress

- Standing one-arm
  shoulderpress

- Side squat, up,
  one-arm shoulderpress

- Standing push-press (thrusters)

- Kneeling shoulderpress

- Standing side laterals

- Standing 'around the world'

- Kneeling side laterals

- Kneeling 'around the world'

- Standing front raise

- Kneeling front raise

- Prone arm raise

- Standing shoulder extension

- Prone shoulder extension

- Stationary lunge rowing

- Kneeling rowing (one knee)
  (one leg on BOSU,
  one foot on floor)

- 3-point rowing (narrow/wide)

- Stationary lunge back fly

- Kneeling back fly

- 3-point back fly
  (same position as rows)

- Prone back fly
  (prone, feet on floor)

- Standing biceps curl

- Lunge with biceps curl

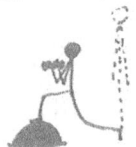

UPPER BODY EXERCISES

- Stationary lunge w. triceps kick back

- 3-point triceps kick back

- Incline triceps extension

- Cross-body triceps extension, bridge position

- Reverse plank, shoulder-stability, bridge position

- BOSU triceps dip

- Chest press, bridge position

- Chest fly, bridge position

- Unilateral fly, bridge position

- Push-up (hands on BOSU)

- Push-up with leg variations

- Push-up, askew (one arm up, one down)

- Push-up, travelling

- Push-up, straddle (legs wide)

- Push-up with BOSU 'dome side down'

- Push-up, rocking, 'dome side down'

- Decline push-up, push-up, feet on the BOSU

CORE EXERCISES

- Ab curl, straight legs

- Ab curl, bent legs

- Boxer crunch
  (ab curl, hands under chin)

- Kick crunch
  (knees bent, kick one leg up)

- BOSU unilateral ab curl test
  (one leg bent, one straight; hand
  to foot). Max. number in 60 sec.

- Knee up (supine open and tuck)

- V-sit (isometric)

- Rolldown

- Rolldown with rotation

- Oblique curl

- Side-lying
  rotated ab curl

- Side-lying lateral flexion

- Side-lying oblique crunch

- Reverse crunch hip-raise

- Reverse crunch toe-tap
  (toe touch down)

- Crunch (double crunch)

- Supine toe-tap, bent legs

- Supine one leg dip,
  (forearms on floor)

- Dying bug (supine)
  (one arm-leg down)

- 'Bicycling' crunch

- Alternating superman:
  all fours, arm-leg lift,
  toes on floor or off floor

- Alternating superman:
  plank, hand on BOSU
  plank, hand on floor

- Superman (hold)

- Prone 'flutter',
  'swim'

CORE EXERCISES

- Back extension

- Hip extension

- Back extension,
  (arms and legs, hold)

- Plank – hands on BOSU

- Plank – toes on BOSU

- Spider – plank
  (start: prone on BOSU, arms and
  legs out, push off and hold, so
  the torso no longer touches the
  BOSU)

- Side plank

- Side plank with rotation

- Side-lying balance,
  support on forearm on floor

- Side-lying balance

- Kneeling balance,
  toes on floor,
  toes off floor

- Kneeling deadlift balance

- Kneeling balance
  with rotation

- Standing balance,
  feet together (start feet wide)

- Standing balance, eyes closed

- Single-leg balance
  (yoga-positions)

- Single-leg balance,
  eyes closed

- T-balance

- Standing single-leg balance,
  w/swings, circles and
  figure eights.

CHAPTER 10 | COOLDOWN

Cooling down is often 'forgotten', but should not be; it is important physiologically and mentally:

When you continue too move your legs, the heart rate is gradually lowered, and the blood is pumped up and back to the heart, this can prevent dizziness.

It is a nice conclusion to workouts; you feel well, become relaxed and prepared for stretching.

The heart rate should be lowered to 50-60 % of maximal heart rate before lying down on the BOSU or the floor for stretching or relaxation.

For BOSU cardio workouts you should always include a cooldown, e.g. use the warm-up activities and progressions in reverse order:

Lower intensity gradually by going from travelling movements to stationary movements and from large range of motion movements to smaller movements.

Slow music and movement tempo down gradually.

You are then ready for stretching or relaxation.

For BOSU strength training workouts of moderate intensity without cardio training, the cooldown could be limited to some standing stretching for the major muscle groups.
Tip: If you keep the body moving slowly and let the movements flow into each other, you will experience 'rhythmical stretching'.

Standing balance work on the floor can also be included as part of the cooldown:

Single-leg balances, on the whole foot or on the toes; lift the free leg outward, forward or backward.

Single-leg stretches, eg. standing thigh or hipflexor stretch on one leg.

The cooldown is completed – the heart rate is lowered to the same rate as before the workout – during the final stretching or relaxation.

DURATION
Cooldown duration depends on the workout intensity and target group. The cooldown following moderate intensity workouts is normally approximately from 3-5 minutes up to 10 minutes after higher intensity workouts.

CHAPTER 11 | FLEXIBILITY

For a relaxing mindful conclusion to the workout include a series of easy stretches for the major muscle groups; focus on the muscles, that are generally tight, eg. calves, hamstrings, hip flexors, thigh muscles and chest (Appendix, TBX).

During stretching focus on deep, slow breathing; preferably through the nose. At the same time relax; let go of tension in the muscles.

Stretches can be of long or short duration depending on the goal. Intense stretching is not necessary; for an easy stretch hold each stretch for 15-30 seconds:
In general fitness the primary goal is to maintain mobility, a functional range of motion.

If time permits and if needed, you can hold the stretches for longer. For increased flexibility hold the stretches for longer than 30-60 seconds. Longer stretches induce a deeper relaxation.

Most stretches can be performed standing, seated or lying on the floor or the BOSU.
The BOSU can be used for seated or lying positions; it is soft and very comfortable, however in the lying positions – as the BOSU is only 8-10 inches in height – the head, arms and legs are on the floor, which may feel uncomfortable.

DURATION
Stretching after BOSU-workouts: Approximately 5-15 minutes.

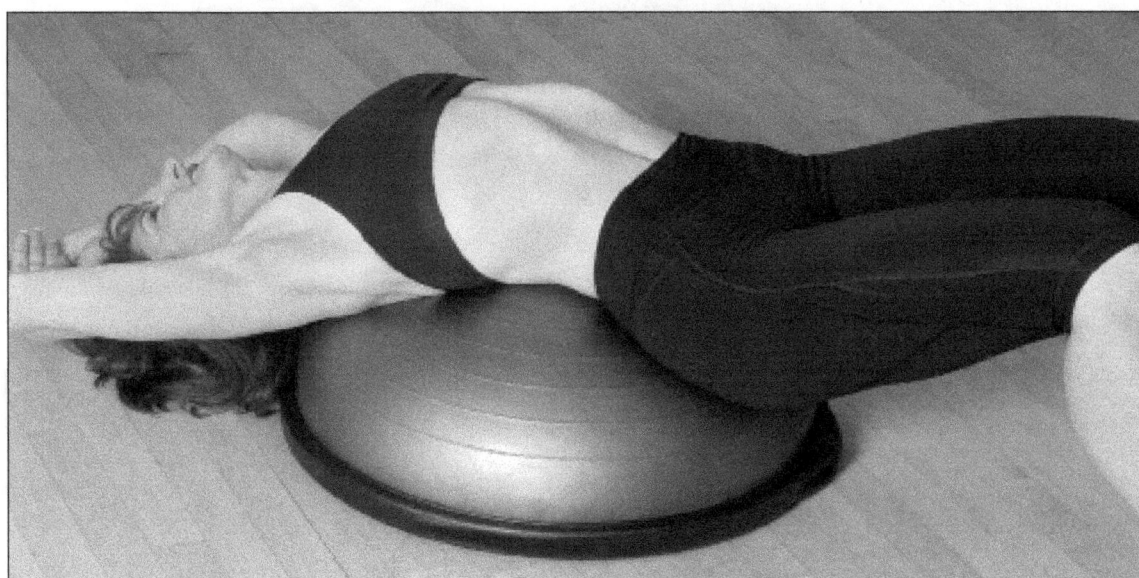

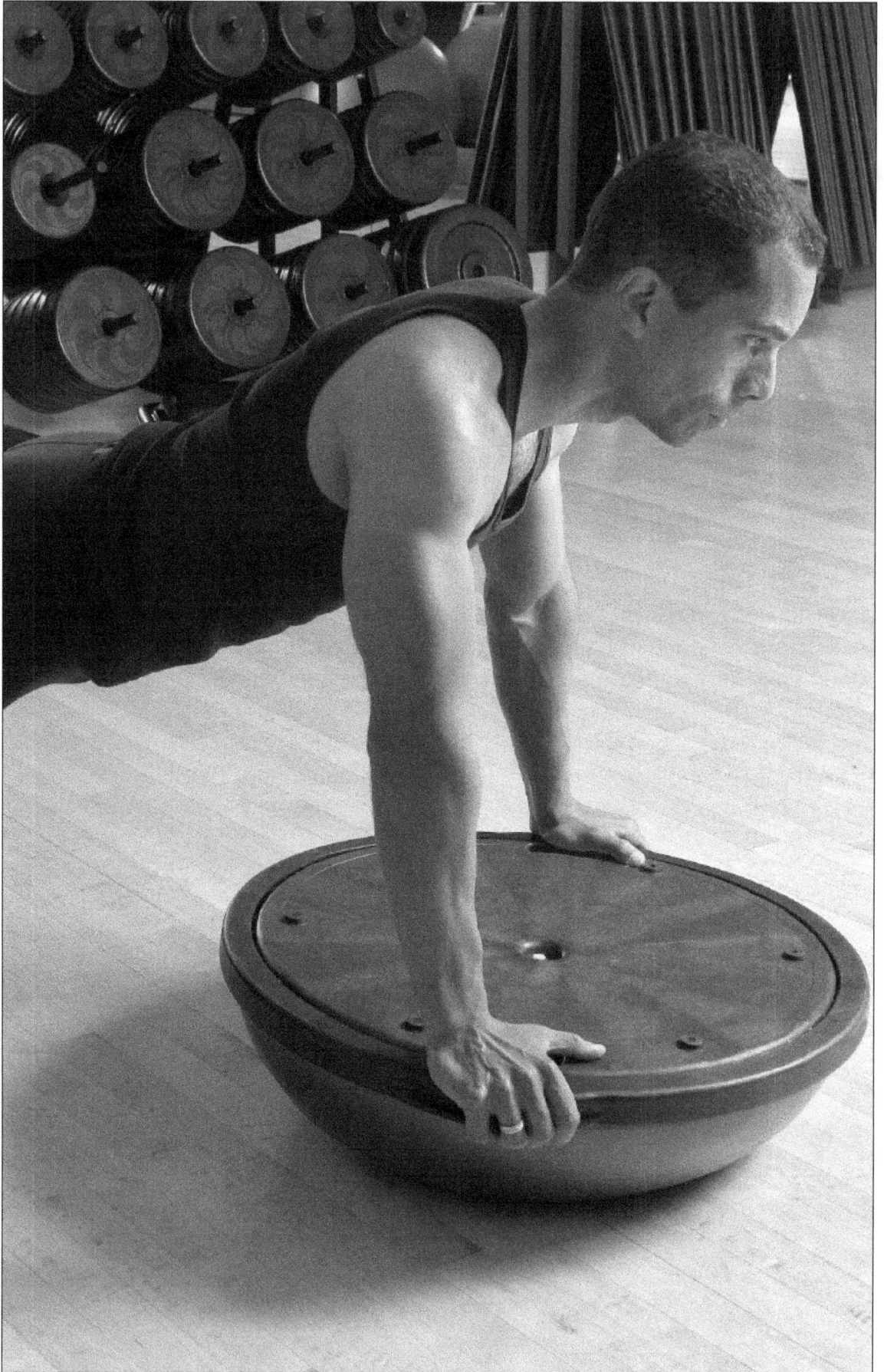

CHAPTER 12 | METHODOLOGY

BOSU instruction is similar to other group exercise and one-on-one instruction, so this chapter is limited to a rundown of the most important and specific principles.
Other books on Group Exercise and Fitness cover the basic principles of exercise instruction.

Before BOSU workouts make a general and flexible plan:

- **Duration**, total duration and duration of each part of the workout: Warm-up, cardio, strength, balance, coordination, cooldown and stretching.

- **Exercises**, exercises throughout the class, suitable for the target group and the workout goal.

- **Intensity**, load and exercise **tempo** – and rhythm (variation).

- **Volume**, 'total load', number of repetitions and sets (weight lifted).

Checkpoints – before class – for safety and workout effectiveness:

- The trainer should come in early to greet and help newcomers feel wellcome and at ease.

- Newcomers should be adviced to wait for the safety cues; *not to* use the BOSU before class intro.

- The trainer should ask about injuries (or beforehand in private) and remind everybody to ask for help if needed during class.

- For newcomers and mixed level group exercise classes, trainers can start with some tips (cues) on proper exercise technique.

- Advanced exercisers seldom need basic cues, but it may still be necessary to correct poor posture or faulty execution.

- Trainers should recommend, that exerciser(s) go at their own pace.

- Trainers should recommend a number of repetitions, for a specific exercise goal, but inform exercisers, that fewer repetitions and rest-pauses are o.k.

Focus points for successful workouts:

BEFORE

Meet newcomers by the door. Introduce yourself and ask for their name (if the exerciser has not already introduced him/her) and say 'hello' or wellcome. Shake hands. Screening: Ask if there are any injuries or health issues to consider.

Introduce/explain the basic position: E.g. Upright posture with the spine, neck and shoulderblades in neutral position. Unlocked, 'relaxed' knees. *Tip: Briefly outline the workout, so the exerciser(s) can prepare mentally and physically.*

DURING

Instruction
Proper technique should be demonstrated and explained clearly and in some detail (not too detailed). Cue exerciser(s) when needed. *Tip: In group exercise; differentiate; show exercises at 2-3 levels.*

Feedback
Keep a keen eye on the exerciser(s) and provide feedback as needed. Move about and assist as needed.

AFTER

Tidy up (lead the way)
BOSU's to the side (racks or depot). Everybody tidies up, BOSU's, mats, weights, etc., after themselves.

METHODOLOGY

Trainers should use several teaching techniques as some learn best by watching, others by hearing and others by feeling the exercise.
If the trainer use both visual, verbal and manual instruction, there is a much better chance of getting the message across faster.
Note: Trainers should be aware, that some exercisers dislike manual instruction, so 'ask for permission'.

VISUAL INSTRUCTION

Visual instruction: The bodylanguage of the trainer including posture and exercise technique. Therefore it is important, that the trainer demonstrates all exercises correctly and in correspondance with the verbal instructions.
If possible, the trainer should, from time to time, discreetly check his/her own technique in the mirror.
The trainer should wear relatively tight-fitting clothes, so exerciser(s) clearly can see, how the exercises should be done.

Note: Exercisers normally mimic trainers closely. So group exercise instructors should first demonstrate, the easiest exercise variation, for the beginners, then more difficult versions, and then go back to the easy version, so beginners know it is o.k. to do the easy version. Advanced exercisers are apt at choosing the appropriate exercise version.

During visual instruction trainers can use gestures and hand signals, cue signs, especially during group exercise warm-ups and cardio work.
If cue signs are used, they should be precise and in time.

Trainers should continually check that exercisers are active and train with good form.

Trainers should have direct eye contact with exercisers most of the time – during group exercise with all participants at least once during the workout – to monitor that the exercisers are well.
Check for signs of excess fatigue.

VERBAL INSTRUCTION

Verbal instruction: Cues and exercise explanations. Also the trainer can use counting or count-downs 8, 7, 6, 5, 4, 3, 2, ...,

Trainers should not talk too much, but save the voice and give the exercisers an opportunity to listen to the body (or the music).

Exercise cues can be general, to several exercisers (a group) at the same time, or specific to one individual exerciser.
Verbal instruction includes:

- Exercise cues, explanations, repetitions and sets. Pep-talk.
- Technique cues.
- Dialogue; questions/answers.

MANUAL INSTRUCTION

Manual, or tactile, instruction:
The trainer uses his/her hands to position or correct the exerciser.
This is an excellent method during fitness resistance training.
A light professional touch gives immediate feedback in relation to correct exercise technique.
If the exerciser cannot feel how the knees should be aligned with the feet, a light toucht on the knees may help. Trainers can use a *hands-on* approach, a touch, or a *hands-off* approach, show how and where to and guide without actually touching the exerciser.

MOTIVATION

Many exercisers attend class or training a couple of times and then stop. It is not unusual as motivation normally dwindles after 4-6 weeks unless something new happens to stimulate motivation.

Trainers can increase motivation:

- Talk to the exercisers before and after the workout or class.
- Make the training easy to follow – no 'insider' talk or terminology.
- Allow beginners to take it easy.
- Create team spirit: Use circuit formats and buddy exercises.
- Use pep-talk and positive music.
- Use several teaching methods.
- Aknowledge exercisers for a good job.

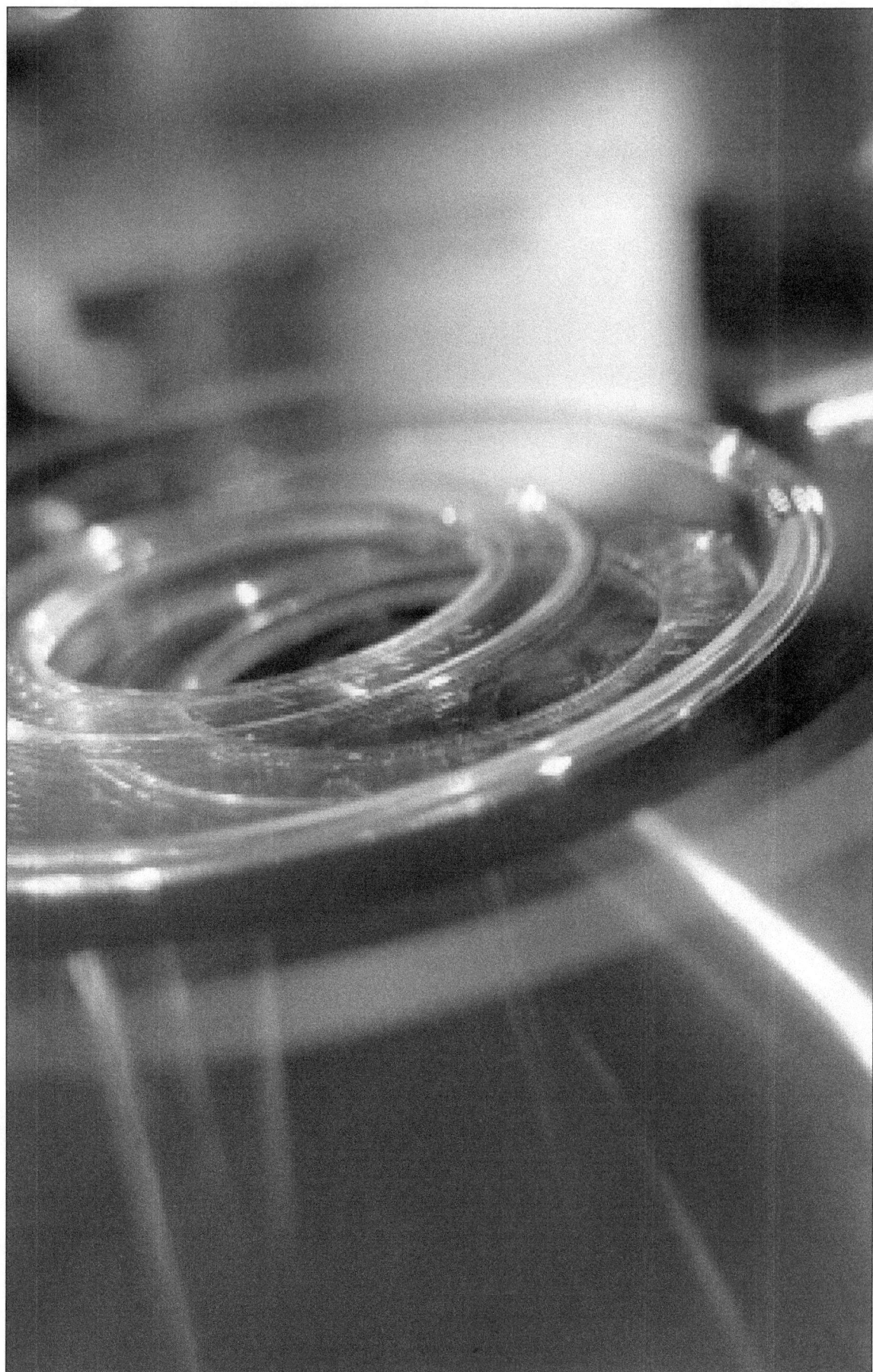

CHAPTER 13 | PROGRAMS

BOSU programs design factors are:

Frequency (workouts per week)

Intensity of the workout

Time, *duration,* of total workout and invidual parts; warm-up, cardio, strength, cooldown and stretching.

The style can also vary according to the goal and the target group

- Age
- Health
- Physique
- Mentality
- Goal

THEME AND STYLE

BOSU group exercise workouts can be designed in many ways. Trainers or instructors can choose specific exercises and build the workout around them or choose a theme and music and then the exercises, e.g.:

1) Establish goal and content.
2) Choose music and theme, style.
3) Choose exercises accordingly.

Workouts *without* music can facilitate concentration and enhance exercise technique focus.

Group exercise without music often fall into these two categories:

Mind body workouts
Exercise with focus on mindfulness. Instructions and feedback in a low to moderate tone of voice. Movements are controlled, even 'silent'. This works well in technical training as well as in relaxation classes.

Sports training
Intense activities, loud commands, shouts and pep-talk, means, that music mainly serves as background music, so it is not strictly necessary. During outdoor activities nature sounds are pleasant 'music'.

To many, however, music is a very important motivating factor and music may well assist the exerciser in perfoming better and for longer. Using music for BOSU-workouts works well.

Music in different genres, with different instrumentation, tempo and rhythm, can create different workout moods and provide variation and hence motivation. Everything from New Age to pop, dance, rock, latin, lounge, funk and techno can be used for different target groups and workout formats.

FORMAT

- Balance training
- Bodytoning
- Core training
- Circuit training
- Interval training
- Agility training
- Hybrid workouts
- Strength training
- Cardio step training

BALANCE TRAINING

A BOSU balance program can be from 5-30 up to 55 minutes. Warm-up, 5-10 min., 5-25 min. stationary and dynamic balancing and 5-15 min. stretching.

A balance program can involve using the BOSU from start to finish or include balance exercises with or without BOSU.

Focus should be on posture and breathing as well as special attention to exercise technique.

Workouts are typically without music, with music at a very low volume (allowing for cues to be heard) or with music; especially for dynamic balances.

BODYTONING

Bodytoning is group resistance training using bodyweight and/or fitness equipment such as tubes, bands, weights, steps and balance equipment.

Focus is on shaping and toning via strength-endurance exercises for all the major muscles of the body. Bodytoning class duration is approx. 55 minutes.

Music tempo is 100-130 BPM (beats per minute).

First posture check. Then a 5-10 min. warm-up: Easy, low-intensity exercises and low impact steps, first without, then with the BOSU. Start on the spot and gradually increase intensity with travelling around and on the BOSU.

Select bodytoning exercises for the major muscles; legs, chest, back and shoulders and arms plus low back and abdominal muscles. Exercise selection should consider agonist-antagonist balance. 8-16 repetitions, or less, of each exercise, and 1-3 sets.

Stretching at the end of class – with or without the BOSU. If you use the BOSU for stretching, then avoid too much 'balance work'; use the BOSU primarily as a bench for seated or lying positions.

CORE TRAINING

In core training focus is on training the center of the body, the core, the inner unit (stabilizing) muscles as well as the outer unit muscles.

Core training workouts can be designed in different formats:

Stationary core training with isometric exercises (holds): Balances, stability exercises and plank positions with or without the BOSU.

Dynamic core training with total body movements, eg. squats with rotations, lunges with rotations and balances. Walking, jogging and running with the torso and limbs in different positions, with rhythm and direction changes.

Dynamic core training could include step training on the BOSU with balancing, travelling and turns.

A mix of dynamic and isometric core exercises is a popular option.

Core training should include a cooldown with easy stretches for the major muscle groups and mobility moves for the spine; flexion, extension, lateral flexion and rotation.

Stretching can be performed on the BOSU, but without balancing; eg. lying and seated balances.

Workouts can be from 10-30 up to 55 minutes depending on the format (intensity). Include a 5-10 minute warm-up and a 5-15 minute cooldown and stretching section.

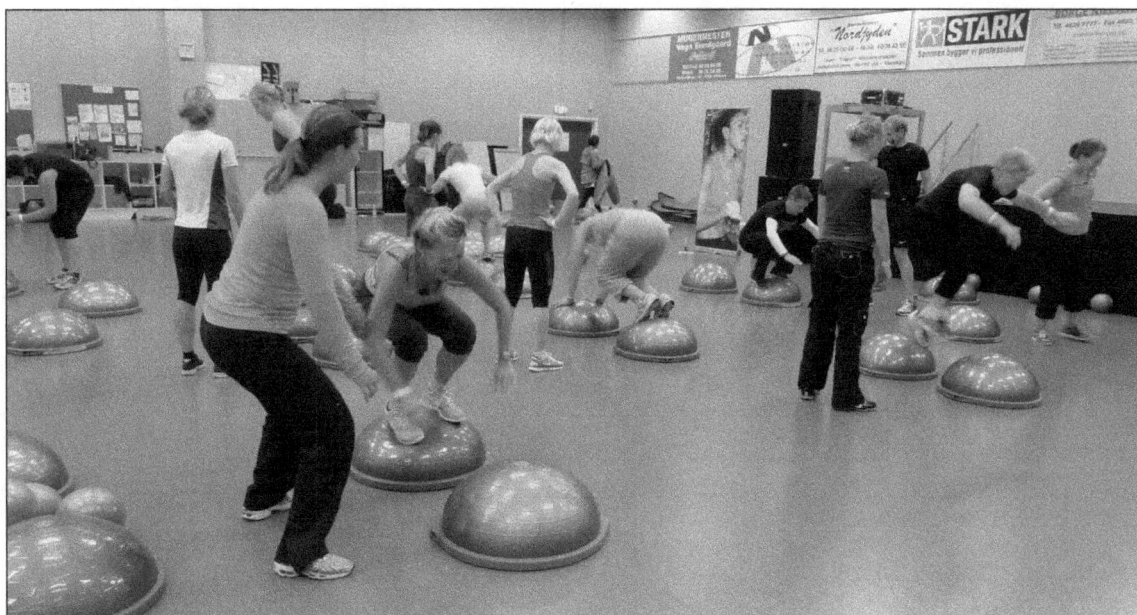

CIRCUIT TRAINING

Circuit training refers to the organization of the workout. The circuit could target cardiovascular fitness, strength or a combination; the latter is the preferred choice for all-round fitness training and general exercise.

Circuit training involves stations with different exercises and equipment. Each exercise, station, is performed for a certain, limited, time period. This makes exercisers work harder; knowing they only have to keep going for a short time. More intense work leads to improved results. BOSU's and other equipment are positioned in a circle format – with mixed cardio and strength stations.

There can be one or two exercisers at each station; two are more fun. There can even be three or more, but this requires more equipment.

You can have from 4-20 stations. Choosing few or many stations gives different possibilities in regard to circuit repetitions (rounds).

The typical time frame of each station is very often ½-1 minute. Station changing time is included in this; you have 5-10 seconds to get set at the next station.

The circuit is repeated 1-4 times.

Total workout duration is 45-55 minutes:
7-15 min. warm-up, 20-40 min. circuit and 5-10 min. of stretching.

You can use pop, dance, techno or rock music with a tempo of 120-140 BPM for circuit training. Optimal tempo depends on the exercise selection.

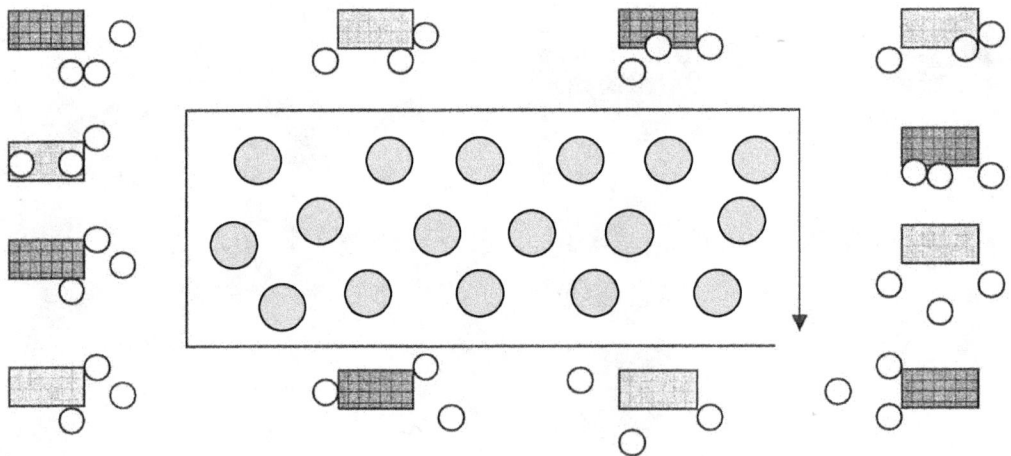

Figure 13.1: BOSU cardio training at the center of the room combined with strength training at stations. E.g. step on the BOSU's in the center of the room, 4 minutes each time, and then one round of circuit training at the stations for 6 minutes (12 stations, 30 seconds each). Repeated 3 times (3 x 10 minutes).

There is a number of possible circuit formats. First of all the BOSU circuit can be designed as a:

Station circuit; a traditional circuit format.
The exercises are performed at stations around the room.
Preferably in a structured set-up, so it is easy to see 1) all of the stations and 2) the sequence of the stations. Each has the same time frame.

The station circuit format allows for:

1) use of many different pieces of equipment/exercises/positions and 2) differentiated instruction; trainers can move around and give individual feedback to each participant.

Unison circuit is set up exactly as traditional group exercise workouts; all exercisers are working out together, in unison, e.g. as in step. Each participant has his or her own BOSU, bench and/or equipment at their own space in the room.

The unison circuit format allows for

1) introduction of new exercises,
2) more advanced exercises,
3) varying duration of 'stations', e.g. 3 min. cardio, 1 min. strength, etc.

These two formats together with the two training modalites cardio and strength makes it possible to create diverse circuits:

- Strength training/unison circuit
- Strength training/station circuit

- Cardio training/unison circuit
- Cardio training/station circuit

- Cardio-strength training/ unison circuit
- Cardio-strength training/ station circuit

- Cardio-cardio training/ unison and station circuit

- Strength-strength training/ unison and station circuit

- Cardio-strength/ unison and station circuit

Tip: Set up the BOSU's in a circle formation or row(s) with the BOSU's close together or apart. Or on lines in a staggered pattern for special circuit training or relay/agility drills.

INTERVAL TRAINING

Interval traning means intermittent training; a number of repetitions of alternating work and active rest periods.

Interval training is optimal for all target groups, because the intensity can be adjusted to suit any level. The determining factor is, that in the interval training work periods the intensity is higher than during continuus work. This means, that *interval training can be performed at a wide range of intensities. It does not have to be of extreme intensity.*

Interval workout
Warm-up, 10-20 minutes.
Intervals, 10-30 minutes.
Cooldown, 5-10 minutes.
Stretching, 5-10 minutes.

Interval training with the BOSU can be high intensity power moves or power stepping (simple steps) with easy low impact moves on the floor during the recovery period.

Interval training can be designed for either aerobic or anaerobic energy system work depending on the goal.

Fitness aerobic intervals

- Long, e.g. 3-5 minutes.
- Repetitions, work/rest ratio, 1:<1
- Sets: 5-7

Fitness anaerobic intervals

- Short, e.g. 15-60 seconds.
- Repetitions, work/rest, 1:2 (3)
- Sets: 8-20

INTERVAL TRAINING ELEMENTS

- **Work interval**
  Exertion, seconds/minutes

- **Recovery interval**
  Activ rest-pause, seconds/minutes

- **Repetition**
  A work and a recovery interval; one cycle

- **Set**
  A series of work and recovery intervals of same or different duration

- **Rest-pause**
  An active rest between sets

WORK AND RECOVERY INTERVALS IN FITNESS INTERVAL TRAINING					
ENERGY-SYSTEM	TARGET HEAR RATE ZONE	WORK INTERVALS		RECOVERY INTERVALS	
		INTENSITY	DURATION	INTENSITY	DURATION
AEROBIC	60-80 % of HRmax	RPE 4-6 moderate	> 3 minutes	RPE 2-3	1:<=1 (1:0,5) Shorter than work interval
AEROBIC/ ANAEROBIC	80-90 % of HRmax	RPE 6-8 hard	½-3 minutes	RPE 2-3	1:1 (1:2) Same as work interval
ANAEROBIC	85-100 % or HRmax	RPE 9-10 very hard	< 30 seconds	RPE 2-3	1:2, 1:3, 1:4 Longer than work interval

Figure 13.2: Work and recovery intervals in fitness cardiovascular workouts. The target heart rate zones serve as a general guide. Rating of Perceived Exertion, RPE, is according to the Borg 10-scale. HRmax is maximal heart rate. (Reebok University Interval Training Guidelines).

INTENSITY AND PERCEIVED EXERTION				
RATING	WORK	SENSATION	BREATHING	SPEECH
1	Very, very light	Inactive	Easy	Normal
2	Very light	Relaxed	Easy	Normal
3	Light	Effortless	Easy	Normal
4	Fairly light	Warm, effortless	Normal	Normal
5	Moderate	Warm, active	Somewhat faster	Almost normal
6	Slight exertion	Some effort needed	Fast	Almost normal
7	Somewhat hard	Strong effort needed	Heavy breathing	Speak with effort
8	Hard	Very strong effort	Laboured breathing	Short sentences
9	Very hard	Very strenuous	Out of breath	Few words
10	Maximal	Near exhaustion	Gasping for air	Talk impossible

Figur 13.3: A modified RPE 10-scale, example. Note, that there are different versions of these 10-scales.

AGILITY TRAINING

Agility is the ability to react and move with speed.
Agility training is for experienced exercisers as it requires a certain level of strength and skill.

The workout can consist of drills aimed at reacting to unexpected signals or cues.
E.g. the trainer can keep cuing new moves, drills or directions.

Agility training is also about the ability to move fast and effortlessly around obstacles; up, down, over, in between, etc.

An agility workout can be designed as an 'obstacle course' with BOSU's in lines or staggered patterns.
Exercises can be running, hopping, jumping and leaping.

Agility workout
Warm up, 15-20 minutes.
Agility work, 10-20 minutes.
Cooldown, 5-10 minutes.
Stretching, 5-10 minutes.

First a thorough warm-up, eg. basic BOSU stepping and easy jogging – and then easy running and hopping.

The actual agility, or sports circuit, program duration should be around 20 minutes maximum in order to keep intensity and concentration.

- Format 1: A relay format with 2-4 rows next to each other.

- Format 2: A station format, a few selected exercises.

- Format 3: A unison format, e.g. modified, easy exercises, for beginners or intermediate level exercisers; walking and jogging.

The BOSU agility course should be organized in advance; away from walls, steps and other equipment.

The participants form one or more lines and move one after the other. Those, who are not active, can jog in place, do push-ups, ab curls a.o.

Agility workouts are fun, but there is an increased risk of injury, because often you are caught up in the drills and forget to be careful. Therefore it is important to minimize the risk of injuries; there must be an adequate warm-up and trainers should provide exercise cues and relevant feedback to make the workout not only enjoyable, but also safe.

The trainer demonstrates or cues exercises, which are performed both to the right and the left. Examples:

- Slalom run between the BOSU's, return (walk) back alongside the row of BOSU's.

- Slalom run backwards between the BOSU's (watch your step).

- Hopscotch, on one leg, slalom, in between the BOSU's (or alongside them).

- Run across the BOSU domes, two steps on each top, two steps on the floor.

- Run across the BOSU's, one step on top, one on the floor.

- Chassé or run sideways along-side the row of BOSU's.

- Run over the BOSU's without touching them.

- Run on the BOSU domes without touching the floor.

- Hop sideways over the row of BOSU's.

- Slalom hop between the BOSU's, jog back alongside them.

- Hop sideways across the BOSU's with an extra hop on the top or on the floor.

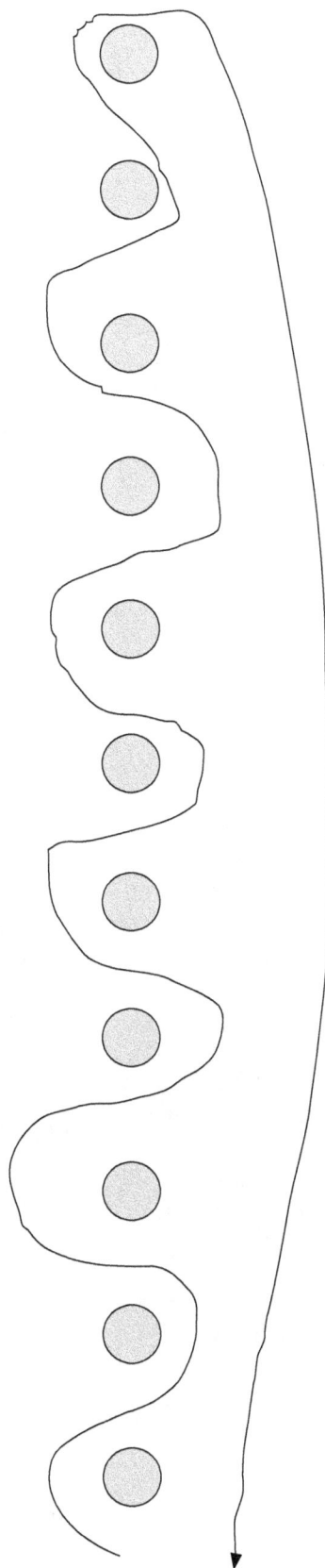

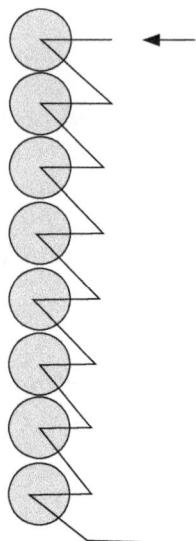

1. Walk/basic step up, left foot leads to the left and right foot leads to the right. After last one jog back to start.

2. Run/basic run up, left foot leads to the left and right foot leads to the right. After the last one jog back to start.

3. Hop up, hold (1,2) walk down (3,4), move to the side, repeat.
   Variation: Add an extra hop on the top. After the last one jog back to start.

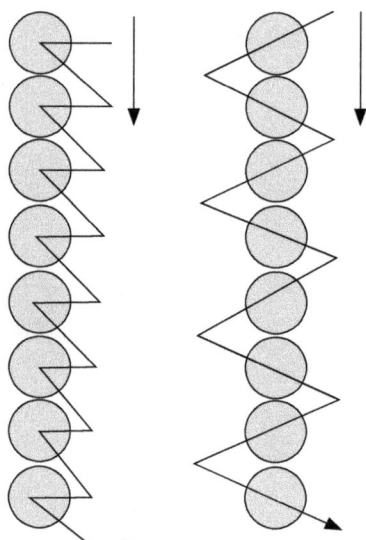

4. Walk/run/jump/hop/sideways up and step down to the same side.
   Advanced: Jump or hopscotch up with ½ or full turn.

5. Walk/run sideways up and across, with power.

6. Walk/run/hop diagonally forward across the BOSU's.

7. Hop laterally over the top and land on the other side. From side to side.

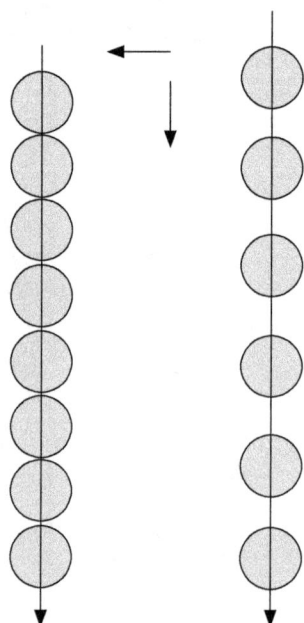

8. Walk sideways or forward on top of the BOSU's.

9. Run sideways or forward on top op the BOSU's.

10. Hop sideways or forward on top of the BOSU's.

11. Jump or hop from BOSU to BOSU with a ¼ or ½ turn.

Have BOSU's side by side or apart.

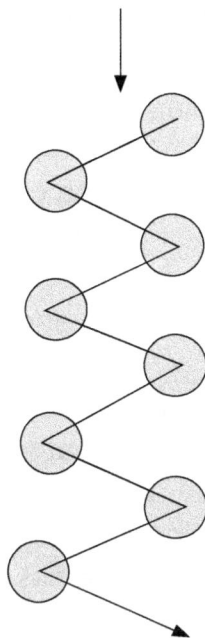

Hop from BOSU to BOSU or have pauses or steps in between.

12. Walk/jog/hop/jump diagonally forward from BOSU to BOSU. Stick/hold for a second on each BOSU. Continue. After the last one, run/return to start.

13. Run forward as if you were racing between tires; the feet down between the BOSU's and up again.

14. Walk up on the top, straddle, step forward to the next BOSU, continue. Same foot leads every time. You can add an extra hop on the top.

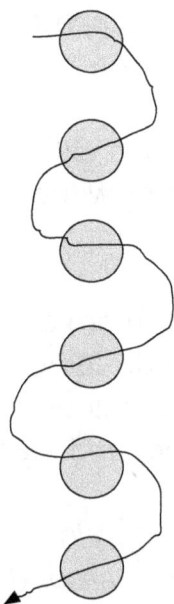

15. Walk/jog sideways over the tops, diagonally forward.

16. Walk/jog sideways over the tops – with extra chassées on the floor.

17. Walk/kneehop sideways over the top. Step up, kneelift, hop change lift the opposite knee, step down on the opposite side. Moving forward.

18. Walk/run/jump sideways over the tops. Perform a floor exercise, e.g. squat, lunge, jack, before returning.

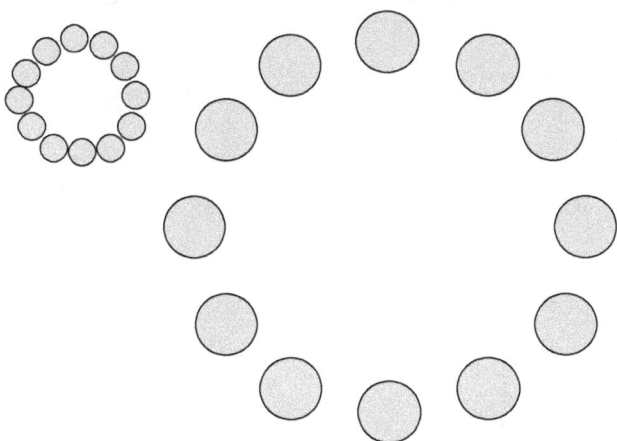

19. Circle formation. BOSU's together or 1-3 feet apart; from the front: Jog up RL, jog down, move sideways and to the right every time. Repeat to the left. Repeat with jumps.

20. Run forward on or over the BOSU's. Run or chassé in slalom forward or backward between the BOSU's. Jump sideways up on/over BOSU's.

HYBRID WORKOUTS

Hybrid training or hybrid classes is a combination of two or more training modalities, e.g. 'spinning and pump' or 'step and strength'.

BOSU work can be combined with many other group exercise modalities, e.g. step, bodytoning, core or balance classes.

A typical structure for hybrid classes is a 10 minute warm up, a 20 + 20 minute activity and 5-10 minutes of cooldown and stretching.

BOSU-work can be either cardio, strength or balance exercises.

After the warm-up you may start with either activity. It depends on which modality you combine your BOSU work with and the goal of the workout.
It is important, however, that the sequence is effective and safe, so you are not complete fatigued by the first part of class, modality number one, so there is a risk of injury during the second part of class, modality number two.

CARDIO – STEP TRAINING

Cardiovascular workouts on the BOSU could be designed as 'step classes' with stepping on the BOSU. Typical class structure is 7-10 min. warm up, 20-40 min. step and 5-10 min. cooldown and stretching.

If you have enough BOSU's, BOSU step classes are great workouts; stepping with an extra dimension. BOSU stepping can be introduced in traditional step classses; e.g. 5-10 minutes during a part of class. *BOSU's, however, are not the best choice for advanced/fast step, which requires attention to choreography.*

You may step in either low or high impact, with or without jogging, hopping and jumping.

You can have more or less stepping and you can do 'aero-step', a mix of steps on the floor (aerobics, jogging, dancing) and step patterns.

Note: The tempo in BOSU stepping should be kept around 120-130 BPM, because the BOSU is higher and more challenging than a step.

RESISTANCE TRAINING

Resistance training with the BOSU is formatted as traditional strength or toning workouts.
Warm-up 5-15 min. Resistance training 10-40 min. and cooldown and stretching 5-10 min.
Resistance training involving the BOSU *and* dumbbells or barbells requires a certain skill level, so:

• Select the exercises carefully to the goal and target group.

• Perform relatively few repetitions, 4-12, per set.

• Sequence your exercises; first the heavy or difficult exercises, then easier, lighter, exercises and finally core training.

For BOSU strength and stability workouts: Perform approx. 6-12 repetitions and 1-3 sets.

The tempo should be moderate to maintain proper technique.
Note: Advancers exercisers may perform with speed with control.

BOSU resistance workouts can include dynamic as well as isometric exercises.

The exercises can be isolations for one muscle group at a time or complex, 'functional' exercises; with movements conditioning the body for everyday life and sports activities; many muscles at work.

To ensure balanced strengthening, in the same workout, or during the same week, you should work opposing muscles, agonists and antagonists, e.g.:

- quads and hamstrings
- chest and upper back
- lats and shoulders
- elbow flexors and extensors
- abdominals and lower back

Focus should be on the muscles, that needs strengthening, e.g. upper back, posterior deltoids, elbow extensors, glutes, hamstrings, abdominals and lower back muscles.

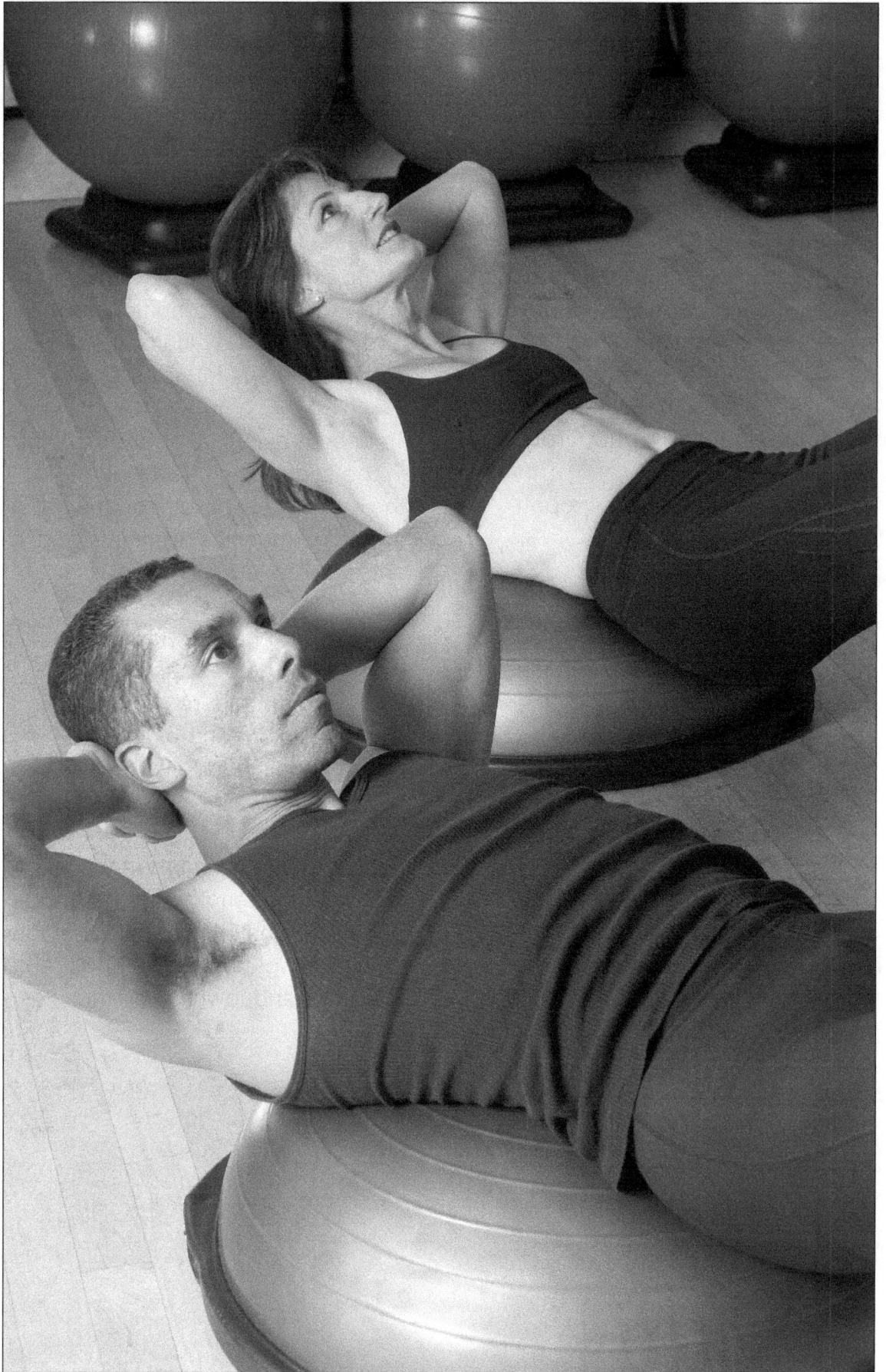

CHAPTER 14 | EXERCISES

Chapter 14 has a table of BOSU strength and stability exercises. To limit the number of exercises, only the basic exercises and more common variations are shown. They are accompanied by text describing further exercises and variations.

Some of the exercises are easy, others are difficult. For some of the exercises there is a note telling if it is one or the other, but not all as several factors contribute to this, which makes exact classification difficult.

Exercise selection should be based on 1) knowledge of anatomy and physiology, sports science and psychology and 2) the health and fitness of the exerciser and 3) goal.

Most exercises can be altered by using one or both arms or legs and by changing the position of the arms, legs or torso.
Most exercises can be made more difficult by gradually increasing the degree of balance work by decreasing the base of support, eg. the feet on the floor or only the toes.

Before working out: The exercises in the book are for healthy exercisers. It is recommended, that anyone new to BOSU training gets help from an experienced BOSU trainer when first starting out.

The BOSU is ideal for rehabilitation work, but this should be under the supervision of a physiotherapist or trainer with special skills.

Standing balance
on both legs

Eyes open

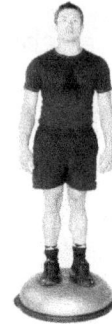

Standing balance
on both legs

Eyes closed

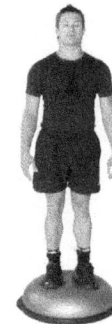

Standing balance
on one leg – single-leg balance

Eyes open

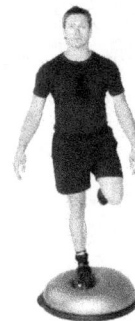

Standing balance
on one leg – single-leg balance

Eyes closed

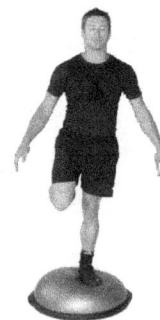

TECHNIQUE	NOTE	VARIATION
Stand on the top. Feet hip-width apart. Erect posture. Look straight ahead. Contract the core muscles. Arm position is optional. Hold the position, eg. 1-3 minutes.	Focus your gaze on a fixed object, so it is easier to keep the balance. The exercise is harder with the feet together and easier with the feet wider apart.	Do squats or single-leg exercises: **Standing hip flexion** Lift one leg forward. **Standing hip abduction** Abduct one leg to the side. **Standing hip extension** Lift one leg backward.
Stand on the top. Feet hip-width apart. Erect posture. Eyes closed. Arm position is optional. Hold the position, eg. 1-3 minutes.	Progress by having one eye closed. The exercise is harder with the feet together and easier with the feet wider apart.	Different arm/leg position.
Stand on one leg on the top. Center the foot on the top. Erect posture. Look straight ahead. Arm position is optional. Hold the position, eg. 30-180 seconds.	Focus your gaze on a fixed object, so it is easier to keep the balance.	Different arm/leg position. E.g. yoga 'tree pose' with the leg externally rotated with the foot on the inner thigh of opposite leg. Free leg movements; e.g. swings or figure-eights. Move, bend and extend, the working leg (1-leg squat).
Stand on one leg on the top. Center the foot on the top. Erect posture. Eyes closed. Arm position is optional. Hold the position, eg. 30-180 seconds.	Progress by having one eye closed.	Different arm/leg position. Perform different movements with the free leg. Bend the working leg.

EXERCISE

Standing balance
on both feet

Bend and extend the neck.
Look down and up (or straight
ahead)

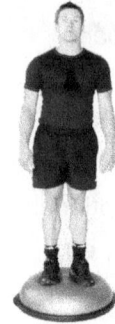

Standing balance
on both feet

Head to the side, neck
lateral flexion, right and left

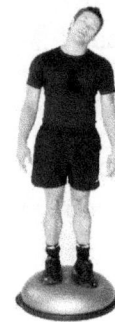

Standing balance
on both feet

Turn the head, neck rotation,
right and left

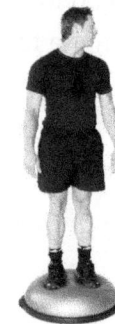

Standing balance
on both feet (or on one leg)

Upper body movements

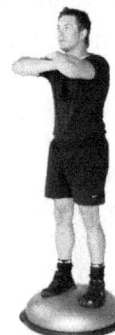

TECHNIQUE	NOTE	VARIATION
Standing on the top. Feet hip-width apart. Erect posture. Look up and down for additional stability work. Contract the core muscles. Arm position is optional. Hold the position, eg. 1-3 minutes.	The exercise is harder with the feet together and easier with the feet wider apart.	Different arm/leg position. On one or both legs. With open or closed eyes.
Standing on the top. Feet hip-width apart. Erect posture. Sidebend the head (neck) to the right and left for additional stability work. Arm position is optional. Hold the position, eg. 1-3 minutes.	Keep the neck in neutral position; sidebend the neck straight to the side, do not move the head forward. The exercise is harder with the feet together and easier with the feet wider apart.	Different arm/leg position. On one or both legs. With open or closed eyes.
Standing on the top Feet hip-width apart. Erect posture. Turn the head to the right and left for additional stability work. Contract the core muscles. Arm position is optional. Hold the position, eg. 1-3 minutes.	Keep the neck in 'neutral position'; turn the head straight to the side, do not move the head forward. The exercise is harder with the feet together and easier with the feet wider apart.	Different arm/leg position. On one or both legs. With open or closed eyes.
Standing on the top. Feet hip-width apart. Erect posture. Look straight ahead. Contract the core muscles. Perform various upper body movements. Hold the position, eg. 1-3 minutes.	The exercise is harder with the feet together and easier with the feet wider apart.	Different arm/leg position. On one or both legs. With open or closed eyes.

Squat

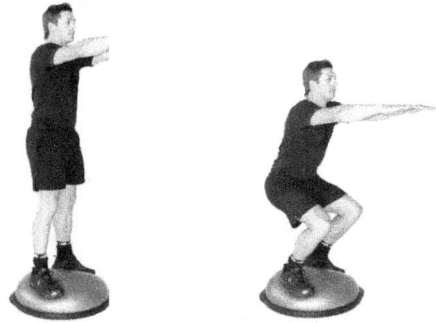

Squat, deep (full squat)

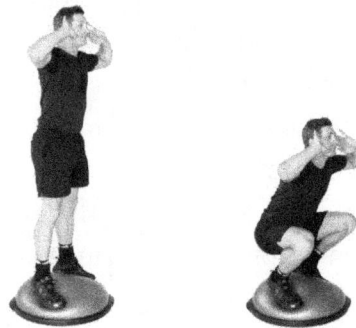

Squat with rotation

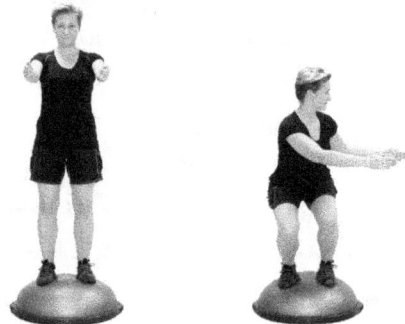

Sumo squat (legs wide)

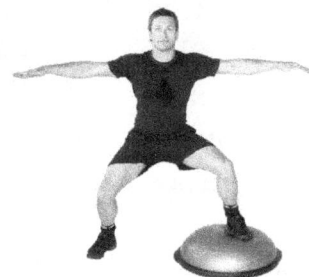

TECHNIQUE	NOTE	VARIATION
Standing on the top. Feet hip-width apart. Erect posture. Look straight ahead. Arm position is optional. Squat: Bend the legs and extend the legs.	Spine in neutral position. Look straight ahead, not up or down. Squats can be performed dynamically or isometrically; holding the position, eg. for ski fitness workouts – hold in different positions.	**Squat with abduction** Squat down. Straighten, extend, the legs, and lift one leg out to the side, abduct. Repeat or change legs. **Squat with hip extension** **Squat with kneelift/kick** **Squat with jump and stick**
Standing on the top. Feet hip-width apart. Erect posture. Look straight ahead. Arm position is optional. Bend the legs and go as low as possible without loosing control and balance. Extend the legs.	Spine in neutral position. Look straight ahead, not up or down. Squats can be performed dynamically or isometrically; holding the position, eg. for ski fitness workouts – hold in different positions.	Different arm/leg position. Different range of motion, 1/4, parallel, full squat. With or without resistance, eg. dumbbell, barbell, medicine ball, kettlebell.
Standing on the top. Feet hip-width apart. Erect posture. Look straight ahead. Arm position is optional. Bend the legs and at the same time rotate the torso to one side. Extend the legs, return. Repeat other side.	Spine in neutral position. Look straight ahead, not up or down. Knees and feet aligned, throughout the exercise; avoid twisting the knees, when rotating the torso.	Different arm/leg position. Different range of motion, 1/4, parallel, full squat. With or without resistance, eg. dumbbell, medicine ball, kettlebell.
Standing. One foot on the top, other on the floor. Legs wide, slight external rotation. Erect posture. Arm position is optional. Bend and extend the legs. Repeat. After a set repeat with the other foot on the top.	Spine in neutral position. Look straight ahead, not up or down. Keep knees and feet aligned at all times. Contract the pelvic floor muscles.	Different arm/leg position. Different range of motion, 1/4, parallel, full sumo squat. With or without resistance, eg. dumbbell, barbell, medicine ball, kettlebell.

EXERCISE

Bulgarian squat

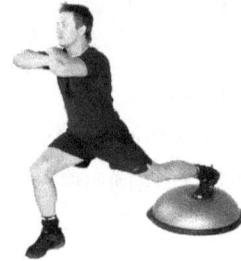

Back lunge
from the top

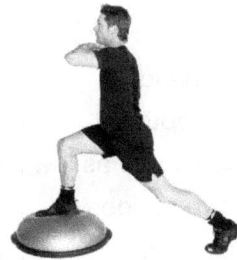

Stationary lunge

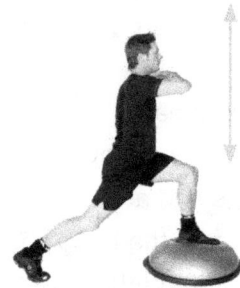

Lunge
from floor to top (front position)

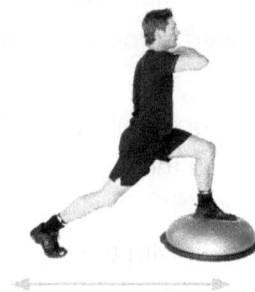

TECHNIQUE	NOTE	VARIATION
Front foot firmly on the floor a lunge step in front of the BOSU. Back foot toes on the top of the BOSU. Bend down into a stationary lunge. Return. Arm position is optional.	Front knee above the foot, it should not move past the foot. Contract the core and keep the torso erect.	Different arm positions. With or without resistance, eg. dumbbell, barbell, medicine ball, kettlebell.
Standing on the top. Feet hip-width apart. Lunge one leg back and down; ball of the foot on the floor, heel lifted, knee bent. Bodyweight centered. Contract top leg and step up again. Repeat with opposite leg	Back heel is lifted off the floor; avoid overstretching the achilles tendon. Knees and feet aligned; avoid twisting the knees. Perform the exercise with control.	**Back lunge with kneelift** From the top: Lunge back (back heel lifted). Push back with the top foot, lift the knee, bodyweight now over supporting back leg. Lunge forward and step back up with the lead leg. Repeat. After a set repeat opposite.
Feet hip-width apart. Front foot on the top of the BOSU. Back leg a lunge step behind, toes on the floor. Stay in this position. Bend the legs, lower, and extend, go back up. Repeat. After a set repeat with the opposite leg in front.	Easy lunge-version; stationary. Legs hip-width apart: Avoid having the feet too close – as walking on a line – as it is more difficult, unless the exercise is a variation for experienced exercisers.	Different arm positions. With or without resistance, eg. dumbbell, barbell, medicine ball, kettlebell.
Stand behind the BOSU. Feet hip-width apart. Lunge forward; front foot on the center of the top, front knee above the ankle. Back heel lifted. Bend the legs. Push back with the top foot, step back. Repeat opposite leg.	Perform as a combination exercise, e.g.: Multilunge: Lunge forward (up), back, to the side. Legs hip-width apart: Avoid having the feet too close – as walking on a line – as it is more difficult, unless the exercise is a variation for experienced exercisers.	**Sidelunge** Stand on the floor by the side of the BOSU. Lunge laterally, foot closest to the BOSU lunges up. Push back. Return. Repeat. After a set repeat with the opposite leg; start from the opposite side of the BOSU.

Overhead lunge
with BOSU

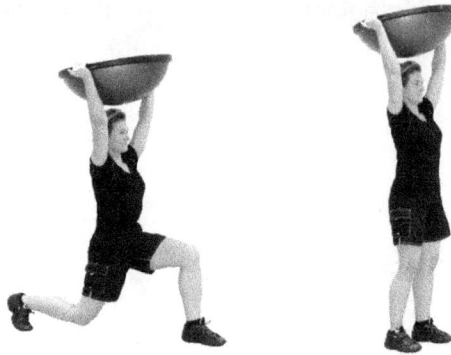

Deadlift with press
with BOSU

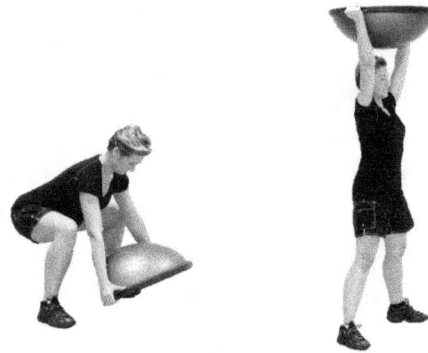

Rumanian one-leg deadlift
with BOSU

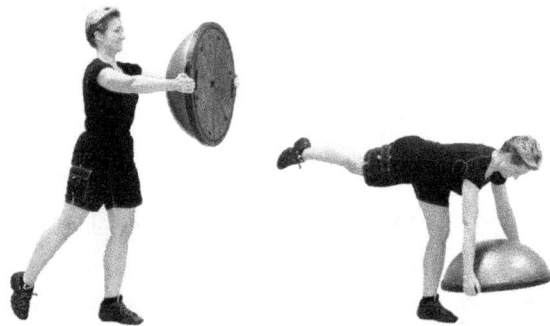

Standing rowing
with BOSU

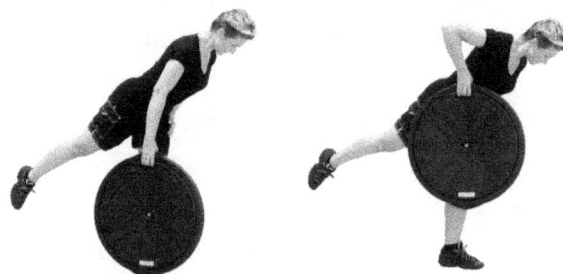

TECHNIQUE	NOTE	VARIATION
Standing. Feet hip-width apart. Hold a BOSU overhead. Lunge forward. Land with the front foot firmly on the ground. Knees bend, 90 dgr. Front knee above the ankle. Back heel is lifted. Push back, return to start. Repeat opposite leg.	For intermediate to advanced exercisers. Contract the core and keep the torso erect. Keep the neck in neutral position and look straight ahead.	Lunge forward with the front foot landing on a BOSU or a step bench. With a barbell instead of a BOSU.
Standing. Feet hip-width apart or wider. Keep the back straight during the entire movement. Hold the BOSU handles and lift the BOSU up and press it overhead. Return; bend the legs well and contract legs and core.	For intermediate to advanced exercisers. Contract the core and keep the spine in a neutral position.	**Swing** For advanced exercisers. Movements with a swing. Requires core control and good technique.
Standing. Feet hip-width apart. One leg behind with the toes on the floor or lifted. Bodyweight over the front leg. Contract the back of the body. Hold the BOSU. Tip forward to a T, scale position. Return up. Repeat. After a set, repeat other leg.	For intermediate to advanced exercisers The free leg can touch lightly on the floor between each repetition or keep the leg lifted off the floor. 6-12 repetitions on each leg.	Different arm/leg position. The BOSU can be held in front of the torso or over the head.
Standing in a scale position, core muscles contracted. Hold BOSU with opposite hand (of the supporting leg). Pull up the arm and BOSU, adduct the shoulderblades. Lower. Repeat. After a set repeat with the other side.	For intermediate exercisers. Keep the back straight. Avoid bending over, letting go of the back and losing stability. 6-12 repetitions on each side.	Arm close to the torso, 'narrow': Latissimus dorsi focus. Arm to the side, 'wide': Rhomboid focus. Toes on the floor or lifted for a balance position.

Push-up
hands on BOSU

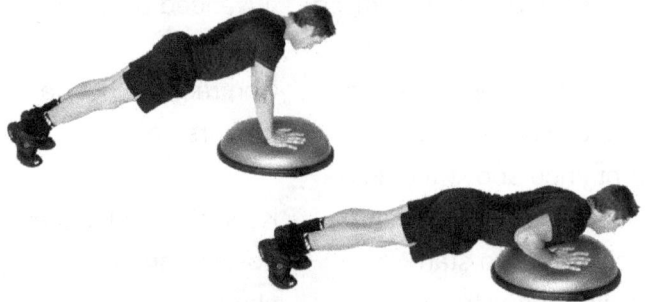

Push-up
hands on BOSU
'dome side down'

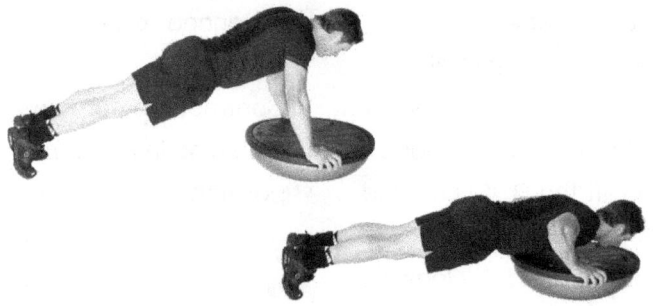

Push-up
feet on BOSU

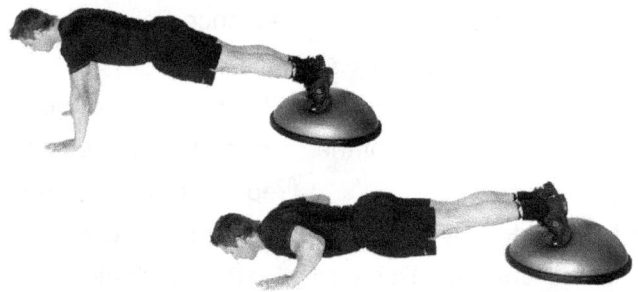

Push-up
feet on BOSU
'dome side down'

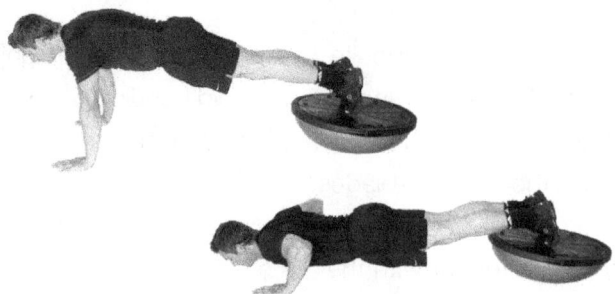

TECHNIQUE	NOTE	VARIATION
Hands on the BOSU. Hands below shoulders. Toes on the floor. Contract the core and keep the body in a straigh line. Bend the arms, lower the body. Extend the arms and push up, return.	Can be performed with *travelling* from one side to the other side. Start: Do an asymmetrical push-up, then both hands on the BOSU, push-up, or continue directly into another asymmetrical push-up on the other side.	**Asymmetrical push-up** One hand on the BOSU, the other hand on the floor. After a set, change side. **Cross push-up (4 BOSU's)** Hans and feet each on a BOSU. Put one hand on the floor, do a push-up. Go up. Then another hand or foot etc.
Hands on the BOSU, 'dome side down'. Hands below shoulders. Toes on the floor. Contract the core and keep the body in a straigh line. Bend the arms, lower the body. Extend the arms and push up, return.	Keep the shoulder girdle stable, do not relax and let the shoulder blades slide. Keep the neck in neutral position, tuck the chin in; do not look up or down. Variation: Hold the position and 'run'; **mountain climber.**	**Burpee push-up** 1. Bend forward, hands on the BOSU. 2. Legs jump back. 3. Feet out. 4. Bend the arms. 5. Extend the arms. 6. Feet hop in. 7. Jump forward. 8. Return to upright position. Different arm/leg positions.
Hands on the floor. Hands below shoulders. Toes on top of the BOSU. Contract the core and keep the body in a straigh line. Bend the arms, lower the body. Extend the arms and push up, return.	Keep the shoulder girdle stable, do not relax and let the shoulder blades slide. Keep the neck in neutral position, tuck the chin in; do not look up or down.	Different arm or leg position. **Staggered push-up** Arms in staggered position. Hands in narrow posiion: triceps focus. Hands wide: chest focus. **Circular push-up** A circular movement in the sagittal or transverse plane.
Hands on the floor. Hands below shoulders. Toes on the BOSU, 'dome side down'. Contract the core and keep the body in a straigh line. Bend the arms, lower the body. Extend the arms and push up, return.	Keep the shoulder girdle stable, do not relax and let the shoulder blades slide. Keep the neck in neutral position, tuck the chin in; do not look up or down.	Different arm or leg position. **Staggered push-up** Arms in staggered position. Hands in narrow posiion: triceps focus. Hands wide: chest focus. **Circular push-up** A circular movement in the sagittal or transversal plane.

Prone balance

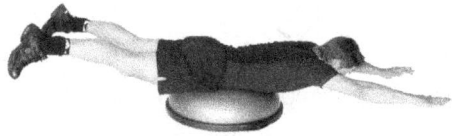

Prone flutter

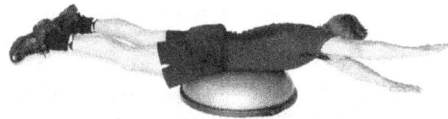

Lower back, hand-to-foot
Prone balance

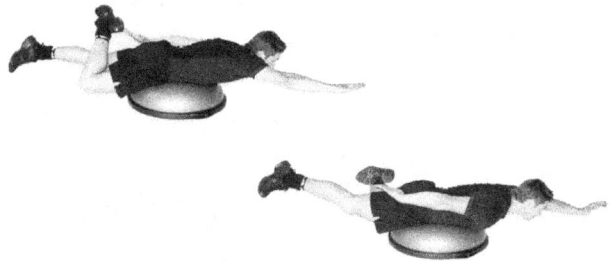

Back extension
Prone on BOSU

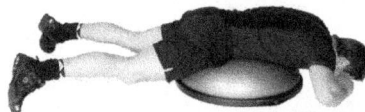

Back extension with rotation

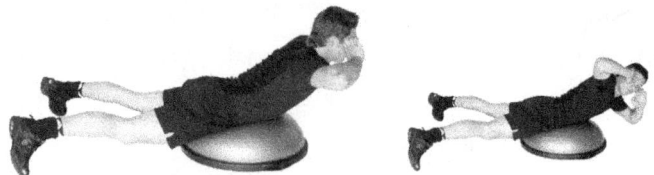

TECHNIQUE	NOTE	VARIATION
Prone on the BOSU. Legs together and lifted off the floor. Arms forward, lifted off the floor, by the side of the head. Keep the neck in neutral position, tuck the chin in. Contract the entire back side and hold the position.	**Dynamic extension** Prone on the BOSU. Lower legs and forearms on the floor. Extend the back and lift the arms and leg. Keep the balance, 2-10 sec. Lower and repeat. **Prone tuck and extend** Perform without pausing.	**Back rock** Prone. Body straight. Arms and legs straight. Lift the torso and lower, lift the legs and lower; the body is rocking like a 'seesaw'. Alternating back extension and hip extension.
Prone on the BOSU. Legs together and lifted off the floor. Arms forward by the side of the head. Move the arms and legs up and down in a (leg) 'crawl' movement, while keeping the balance.	Contract the entire back side of the body and hold the position. Keep the neck in neutral position.	**Hip extension** Prone. Forearms on the floor in front of the BOSU. Legs together. Lift the legs. Lower the legs with control. Repeat without pausing.
Prone on the BOSU. Legs together and lifted off the floor. Arms forward off the floor. Contract the entire back side. Bend the right leg and touch the foot with the left hand. Change hand and leg.	Contract the entire back side of the body and hold the position. Keep the neck in neutral position.	Opposite arm and leg to the side, abduction. Return. Repeat opposite side.
Prone on the BOSU. Hands by the shoulders, temple or forward. Toes (lower legs) on the floor. Extend the back, lift the torso into back extension. Lower with control.	Lower legs on the floor or lifted, supporting only on the toes. With or without torso rotation. Different arm positions.	**Back extension with rotation** Lift and rotate to the side. Lower. Repeat opposite side. **Back extension and sidebend** Lift and sidebend; angle variation. Lower. Repeat other side. **Kneeling deadlift** Kneeling balance, bend hips and knees. Return to start.

Plank
on all fours
hands on floor,
legs on BOSU

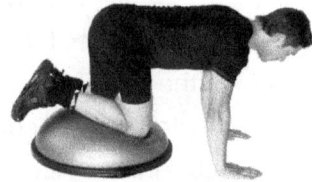

Alternating superman
kneeling
hands on floor,
lower leg on BOSU

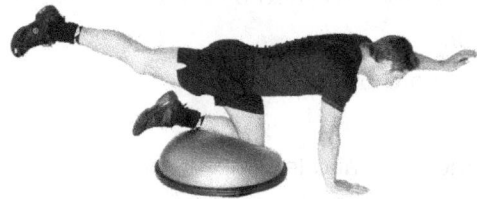

Alternating superman
plank position
hands on floor,
feet on BOSU

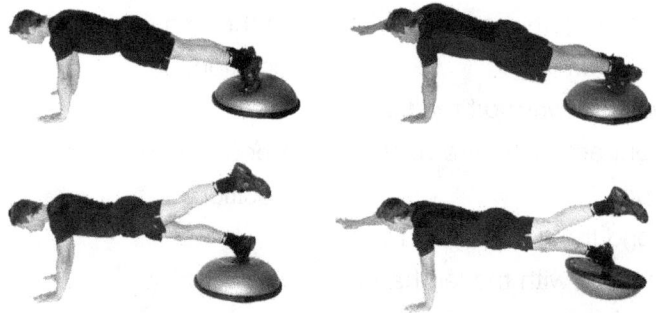

Alternating
superman
plank position
hands on BOSU,
feet on floor

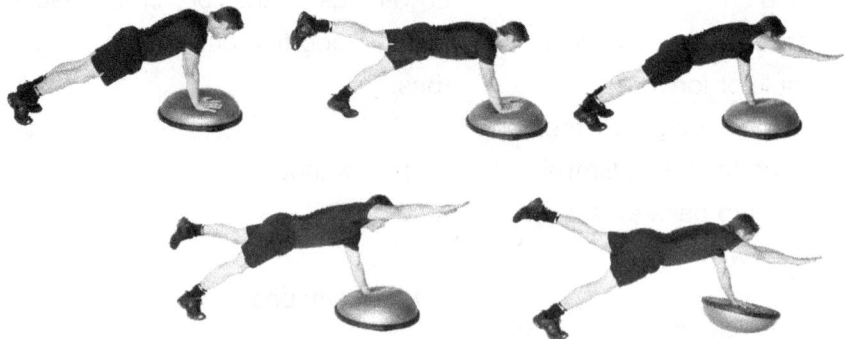

TECHNIQUE	NOTE	VARIATION
On all fours. Lower legs on the BOSU. Hands on the floor. Hands below the shoulders. Contract the core and keep the spine in neutral position. Keep the neck in neutral position. Hold the position.	Keep breathing. Contract the core and keep the spine in neutral position. Keep the neck in neutral position. Watch the wrists; hands directly below the shoulders.	Different arm/leg position. All fours position, hands on the floor, only toes on top of the BOSU. Variation: Lift one leg. On all fours on the top.
On all fours. Lower legs on the BOSU. Hands on the floor. Hands below the shoulders. Contract the core. Spine and neck in neutral position. Lift right arm and left leg to horizontal. Lower. Repeat other side.	Keep breathing. Contract the core and keep the spine in neutral position. Keep the neck in neutral position. Watch the wrists; hands directly below the shoulders.	Different arm/leg position. In top position move the arm and leg to the side. Or move the hand and foot together. **Alternating superman** On all fours on top of the BOSU. Lift the opposite arm and leg alternatingly.
Plank position. Hands on the floor, hands below shoulders. Feet on the BOSU. Contract the core, stabilize. Body in a straight line. Neck in neutral position. Lift one leg or one arm or opposite arm and leg. Alternate.	Keep breathing. Watch the wrists, perform with control. Contract the core and keep the spine in neutral position. Keep the neck in neutral position.	Different arm/leg position. Make circular movements with the arm or the leg. BOSU 'dome side down'.
Plank position. Hands on the BOSU. Hands below the shoulders. Feet on the floor. Contract the core. Body in a straight line. Neck in neutral position. Lift one arme or one leg or opposite arm and leg.	Watch the wrists. Keep breathing. **Asymmetrical plank** Hands on the BOSU. Toes on the floor. Right hand on the floor, left foot out. Left hand on the floor, right foot out. Right hand back up, left foot in, left hand up, right foot in. Repeat.	**Burpee with side jump** 1. Bend down, hands on BOSU 'dome side down'. 2. Legs jump backward. 3.-4. Feet jump out//in. 5. Legs jump forward/right. 6. Legs jump backward. 7. Legs forward. 8. Stand up. Repeat and jump left.

Bridge
bridge position on BOSU

Dynamic or isometric

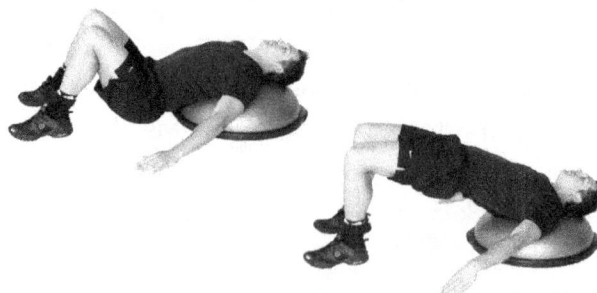

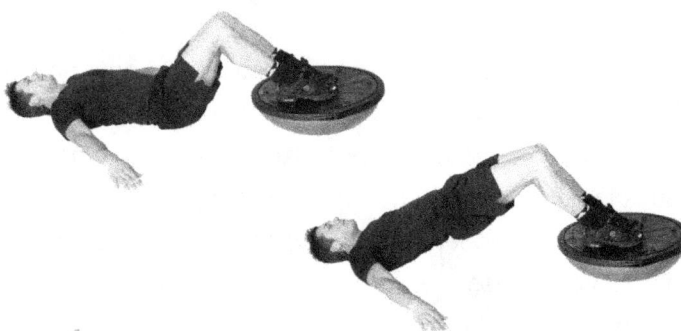

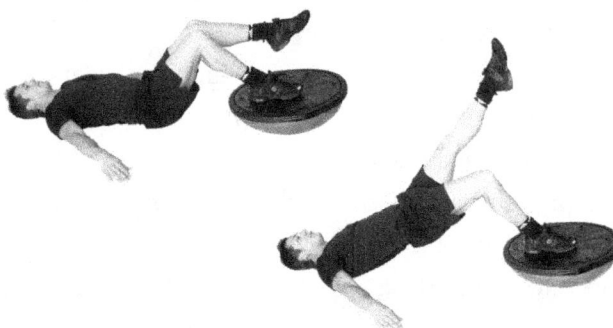

Bridge
bridge position on floor,
feet on BOSU,
'dome side down'

Dynamic or isometric

Bridge on one leg
bridge position on floor,
foot on BOSU,
'dome side down'

Dynamic or isometric

March
bridge position on floor
feet on BOSU,
'dome side down'

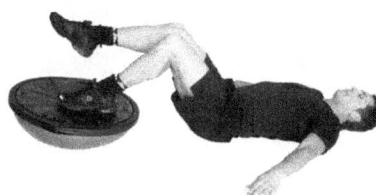

TECHNIQUE	NOTE	VARIATION
Supine on the BOSU. Feet on the floor. Contract the backside of the body and lift the body into bridge position. Hold the position or lower and lift alternatingly.	Support on the upper back, *not* on the neck. Isometric exercise; hold the position and keep breathing. Dynamic exercise; contract and lift, lower with control.	One foot on the floor, the other leg straight and parallel to the floor or bent close by the support leg.
Supine on the floor. Feet on the BOSU 'dome side down'. Contract the backside of the body and lift the body into bridge position. Hold the position or lower and lift alternatingly.	Support on the upper back, *not* on the neck. Isometric exercise; hold the position and keep breathing. Dynamic exercise; contract and lift, lower with control.	One foot on the BOSU. Feet on the BOSU dome.
Supine on the floor. One foot on the BOSU 'dome side down'. Free leg by the working leg. Contract the backside of the body and lift the body into bridge position. Hold the position or lower and lift. After a set, change legs.	Intermediate level. Support on the upper back, *not* on the neck.	Hold the leg, straight or bent, by the opposite leg. Feet on the BOSU dome.
Supine on the floor. Feet on the BOSU 'dome side down'. Contract the backside of the body and lift body into bridge position. Hold the position, hips raised and level. 'Walk' with your feet on top of the BOSU.	Support on the upper back, *not* on the neck.	Different arm/leg position. Feet on the BOSU dome.

Sidelying balance
Lateral balance

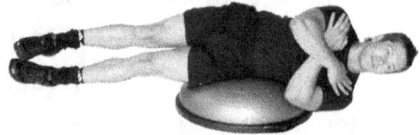

Side plank
Arm on BOSU

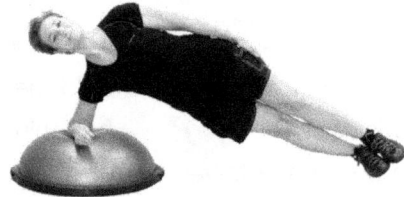

Side plank
Feet on BOSU

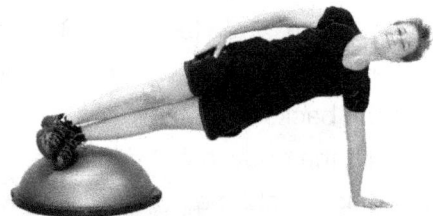

Sidebend
sidelying on BOSU

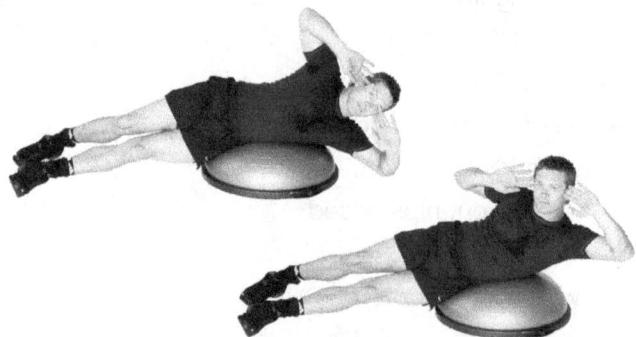

TECHNIQUE	NOTE	VARIATION
Sidelying on the BOSU. Keep the legs straight and together and lifted off the floor. Arms folded across the chest or extended behind the head. Find your balance and keep your body in a straight line.	Contract the core, stabilize and keep the body on a straight line. Keep the neck in neutral position, avoid lifting the head sideways. Keep breathing.	**Sidelying abduction** Lying on the side, support on the forearm, legs lifted. Lift the top leg up and lower to work the abductors and balance. **Sidelying hip flexion, hip extension and 'scissors'**
Sidelying on the BOSU. Forearm or hand on BOSU. Keep the legs straight and together. Feet staggered or on top of one another. Find your balance and keep your body in a straight line.	Contract the core, stabilize and keep the body on a straight line. Keep the neck in neutral position, avoid lifting the head sideways. Keep breathing.	**Side plank with rotation (lateral twisting plank)** Side plank position. Rotate the torso towards the floor and move the free arm under the torso to the back. Rotate the torso towards the ceiling and move the free arm up and to the back.
Sidelying on the BOSU. Forearm or hand on the floor. Keep the legs straight and together. Feet staggered or on top of one another on the BOSU. Find your balance and keep your body in a straight line.	Contract the core, stabilize and keep the body in a straight line. Keep the neck in neutral position, avoid lifting the head sideways. Keep breathing.	Move the top leg; abduction, flexion, extension, circles, figure eights. BOSU 'dome side down'.
Sidelying on the BOSU. Feet on the floor. Legs straight or bent. Legs staggered or together on top of each other. Arm position is optional. Sidebend the torso. Lower with control. Repeat.	After a set change side. Keep the neck in neutral position, avoid lifting the head sideways. Keep breathing.	Different arm/leg position.

Supine balance
Isometric front side work

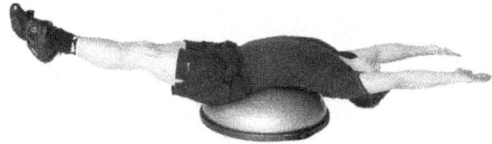

Spider plank

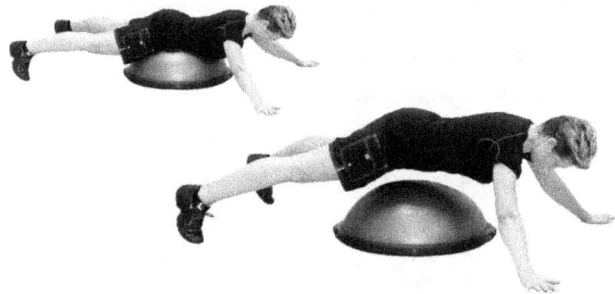

Ab curl
supine on BOSU

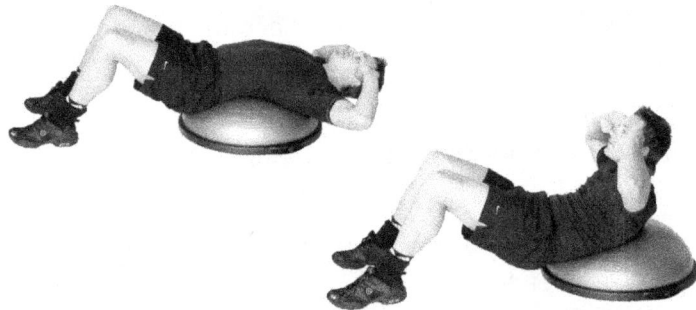

Oblique curl
supine on BOSU

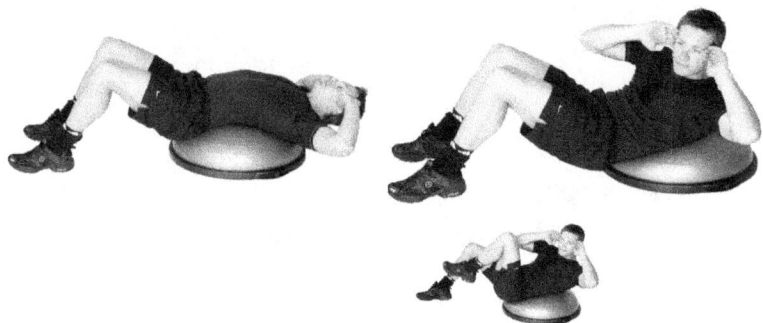

TECHNIQUE	NOTE	VARIATION
Supine on the BOSU. Legs straight and together and lifted off the floor. Arms straight back by the head. Contract the muscles on the front of the body. Keep the body in a straight line and balance. Hold the position.	Keep the neck in neutral position. Contract the abs; avoid hyperextension of the back. Keep breathing.	Tabletop position (legs bent 90 degrees, hip and knee). **Hip lift** Supine in tabletop position. Lift the pelvis slightly. Lower. **Alternating leg drops** Forearms on the floor behind the BOSU. Legs vertical. Lower one leg at a time.
Prone on the BOSU. Arms and legs diagonally to the side. Hands and toes on the floor. Contract the abdominals and lift the body off the BOSU. Keep the body in plank position.	Keep the neck in neutral position. Contract the abs; avoid sagging of the back. Keep breathing.	Different arm/leg position.
Supine on the BOSU. Feet on the floor. Hands on the chest, by the temple or to the back. Contract the abdominals and curl up the torso. Lower with control.	**Ab curl** is upper body flexion. **Reverse curl** is a lower body 'crunch', pelvic tilt. **Crunch** is moving the upper and lower body towards each other. Ab and reverse curl at the same time.	Different arm/leg position. **Straight leg crunch** Ab curl with legs straight. **Kick crunch** Crunch, one leg kicks up. **Boxer crunch** Bend the arms and place hands under the chin to keep the head still; ab curl.
Supine on the BOSU. Feet on the floor. Hands on the chest, by the temple or to the back. Contract the abdominals, curl up and rotate to the side. Lower with control. Repeat to the opposite side.	Repeat the exercise to the same side, e.g. 8-12 reps. Then change side. Or alternate: curl right and left. With or without lifting the opposite leg.	**Lateral ab curl** Curl up in an ab curl and at the same time side bend. Return to starting position. Repeat opposite side. **Ab curl with legs to side** Legs bent, together and to the side. Curl up. Lower. After a set repeat opposite.

Supine bicycling

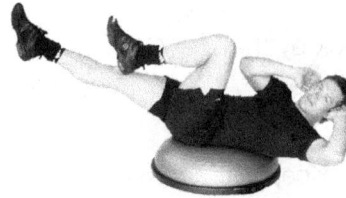

V-sit
Bent or
straight legs

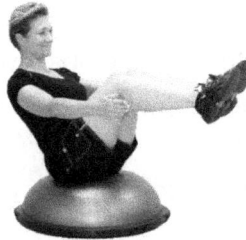 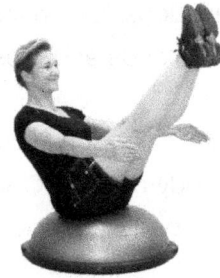

V-sit with rotation

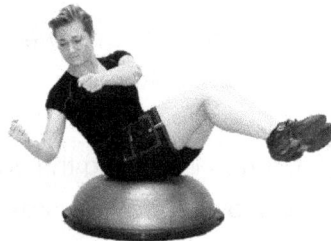 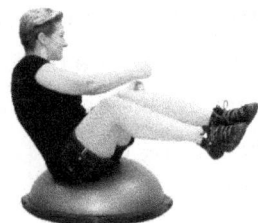

Knee-up

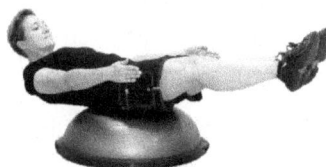 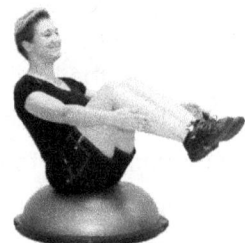

TECHNIQUE	NOTE	VARIATION
Supine on the BOSU. Legs straight. Hands by the temple. Contract the abs, curl up the torso and rotate. At the same time pull in one leg, opposite shoulder and knee towards each other. Return to starting position. Repeat other side.	Intermediate level. Contract the core to avoid hyperextending.	**Alternating leg drop (tap)** Tabletop position; supine, legs bent 90 degr. Lower one leg/foot to the floor. Return. Repeat opposite leg.
Sitting on top of the BOSU. Hips flexed. Legs bent or straight. Contract the core to keep the position and protect the back. Arms forward or to the side. Hold the position.	Intermediate level. Isometric exercise. Start by holding on to the BOSU and bend the legs. Let go, hands away and slowly extend the legs.	**V-sit with support** Sitting on the floor in front of the BOSU with bent legs. The lower back is supported on the BOSU. Contract the abdominals and the hip flexors and crunch to a V-sit position on the floor. Hold. Repeat 2-5 times.
Sitting on top of the BOSU. Hips flexed. Legs bent or straight. Contract the core to keep the position and protect the back. Arms forward. Twist the lower body to one side and the arms to the other side. Alternate.	Intermediate level. Isometric or dynamic exercise. Start by holding on to the BOSU and bend the legs. Let go with the hands and slowly extend the legs.	Different range of motion. With or without a medicine ball, dumbbell or kettlebell in the hands.
Sitting on top of the BOSU. Legs bent or straight. Arms forward. Contract the abdominals and hip flexors and perform a knee-up; crunch and bring torso and legs up/together.	Intermediate level. The exercise can be made easier by making the range of motion smaller. Start by holding on to the BOSU and bend and extend the legs.	Different range of motion. **Crunch** Tabletop position; supine, legs bent 90 degr. Crunch; 'pull' the torso and pelvis towards each other. Lower with control. Repeat.

Bent-over rowing
kneeling on BOSU

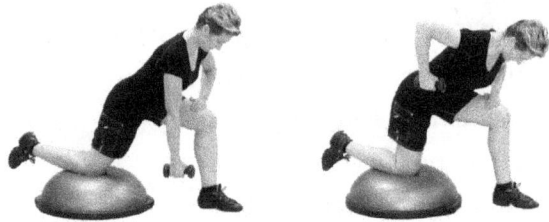

Unilateral chest press
bridge position on BOSU

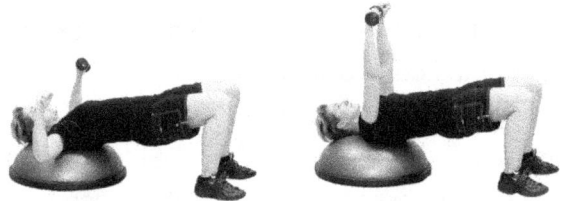

Upper body exercises
standing or kneeling
on the BOSU

Shown here: Around the World
shoulder exercise

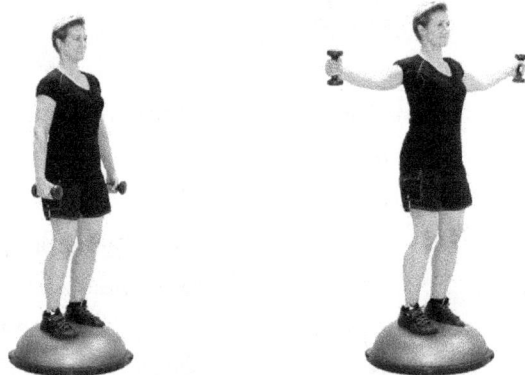

Shoulder girdle work
on the BOSU

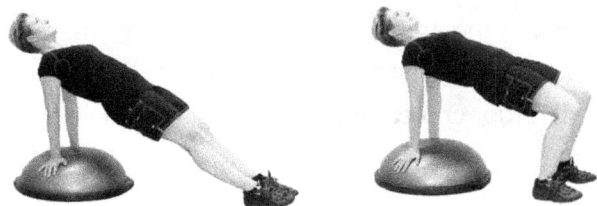

TECHNIQUE	NOTE	VARIATION
Half kneeling on the BOSU. Lower leg on the top, toes on or off the floor. Torso forward. Front hand on front thigh. Contract the core to stabilize. Dumbbell in one hand. Raise the arm to the side, elbow leading. Adduct the shoulder blades. Lower with control.	The exercise can be done with both lower legs on the BOSU and one hand on the floor (three-point support). The exercise can be done as a combination; e.g. rowing and triceps kick back.	**Standing, kneeling or prone back fly** **Rowing,** both arms, 'narrow', elbow to the back, latissimus, or 'wide', elbow to the side, rhomboid focus. **Prone shoulder extension, various angles**
Supine, upper back, on BOSU. Feet on the floor. Arms bent, perpendicular to the torso. Dumbbell in one hand. Extend the arms vertically. In top position move the dumbbell to the opposite hand. Lower both arms. Repeat.	While the arm with the dumbbell is moving, keep the free arm vertical - ready for receiving the dumbbell. The exercise can be done in combination with e.g. chest-press, french press (triceps extension) or chest press and chest fly.	**Chest press (both arms)** With dumbbells or a barbell. **Chest flys** One or both arms, slightly bent, to the side, perpendicular to the torso. Arms retur to vertical above the chest.
Standing on the BOSU. Feet hip-width apart. Arms at sides. Dumbbells in hands. Raise the arms to the side. At horizontal turn palms forward. Arms continue upwards to vertical. Lower the arms in front of the body. Repeat.	Some upper body exercises can be performed in a seated position. It is easier to balance, but the back should be in neutral position, no hunching. Proficient exercisers can combine upper body with lower body movements.	**Front raise, lateral raise, shoulder press, etc.** **Triceps extension,** arms up or to the back (kick back). Supine: **French press.** **Biceps curl, with overhand, underhand or neutral grip.** BOSU 'dome side down'.
Sitting on the BOSU. Hands on the BOSU, fingers point outward or forward. Raise the body and support on the hands and heels. Keep the shoulders down and the body in a straight line. Hold for 2-10 seconds. Lower. Repeat 8-16 times.	For the back side muscles. Keep the neck in neutral; do not drop the head.	**Reverse plank** Straight legs. Heels on floor. Hands, forearms or upper back on the BOSU. Body lifted into reverse plank. **Crab** Reverse plank with bent legs. Hold or walk the feet on the floor.

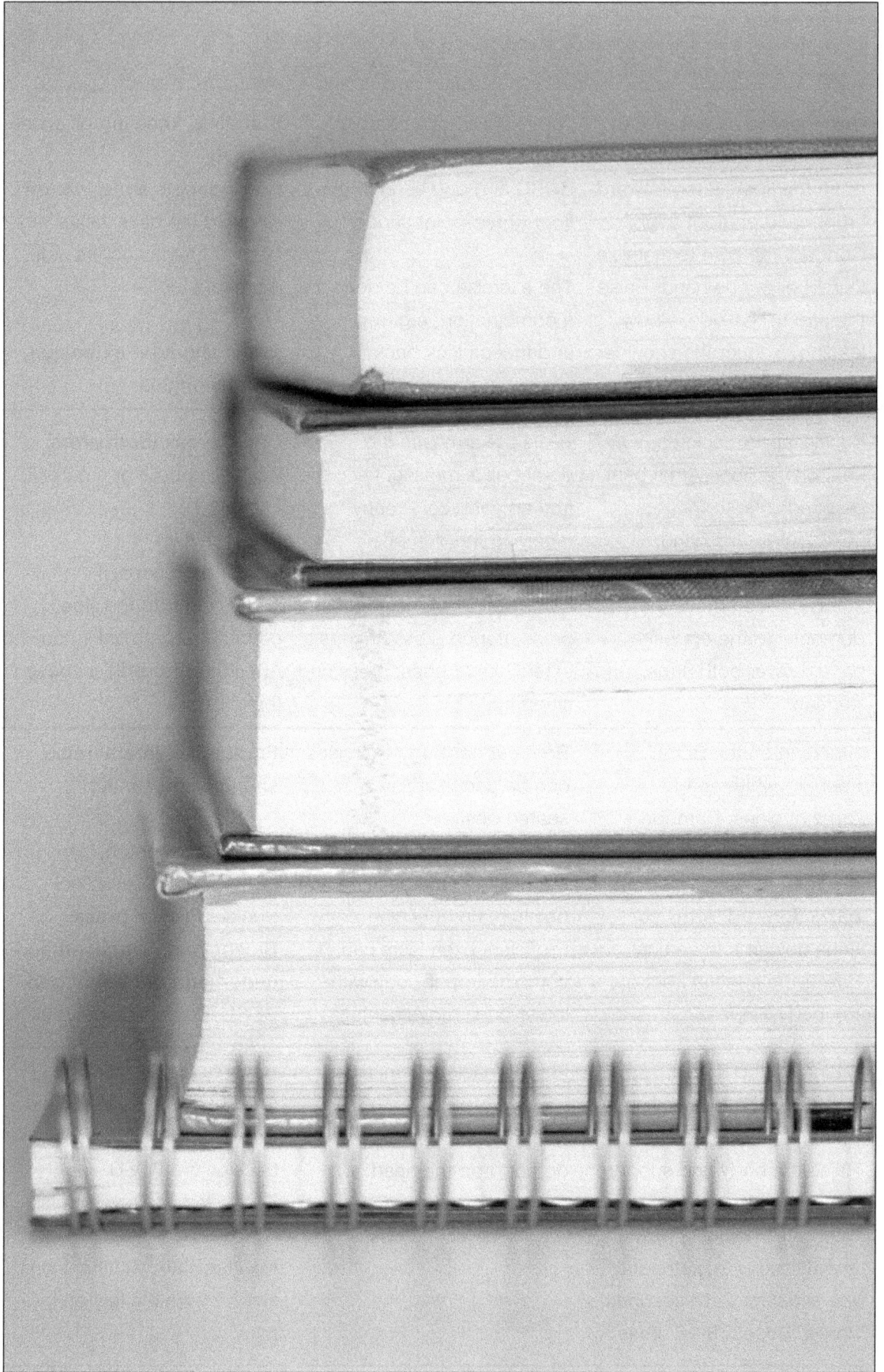

LITTERATURE

BOOKS | RECOMMENDED READING

Blahnik, J, Brooks, D, Brooks, C (2006), BOSU Balance Trainer Complete Workout System.

Gjerset, A et al. (2002), *Idrættens Træningslære, 2. udgave,* GAD København.

Jensen, K (2010), The Flexible Periodization Method, The Write Fit.

McGill, SM (2004), *Ultimate Back Fitness and Performance*, Wabuno Publishers.

Aagaard, M (2010), *Fitness og styrketræning, 2. udgave.* Aagaard.

Aagaard, M (2010), *Resistance Training Exercises.* Aagaard.

Åstrand, P-O et al. (2003). *Textbook of Work Physiology, 4th Edition*, Human Kinetics, Ill.

HOMEPAGES | ADDRESSES

http://www.bodybuilding.com

http://www.chekinstitute.com

http://www.fitnesswellnessworld.com

http://www.ncbi.nlm.nih.gov/pubmed/

http://www.ptonthenet.com

http://www.t-nation.com

http://www.yestostrength.com

GLOSSARY

Ab curl	Abdominal curl. Spinal flexion.
Abduction	Movement of a limb away from the median plane of the body.
Adduction	Movement of a limb toward the median plane of the body.
Aerobic	Utilizing oxygene.
Agility	Moving with ease (sprint, jump and reaction training).
Amplitude	Range of motion, ROM.
Anaerobic	Without sufficient oxygene.
AROM	Active Range Of Motion.
Ballistic stretching	Rapid (uncontrolled) stretching.
BOSU	BOth Sides Utilized. Training equipment.
Cardio	Cardiovascular (training).
Circuit training	Program consisting of stations with different exercises
COG	Center of gravity.
Concentric	Muscle contraction, muscle shortening.
Continuus	Non-stop action (endurance training).
Contraindicated	A contraindicated exercise is a movement, that is not recommended, because it is potentially dangerous.
Coordination	Neuromuscular action; the ability to control the body and limbs, execute movements smoothly and accurately.
Core	Center of the body, inner and outer unit muscles from the pelvic floor to the diaphragm.
Eccentric	Muscle action, lengthening under tension.
Elastic	Resilient. (Elastic bands, variable resistance).
Energy	Capacity to perform work.
Endurance	Ability to bear fatigue. Long duration training.
Explosive strength	Maximal force in minimal time.
Extension	Increasing the joint angle. Straightening.
Flexion	Decreasing the joint angle. Bending.
Frontal plane	Coronal plane, vertical plane dividing the body into front and back sections. Movements to the side.
HR	Heart rate.
Hyperextension	Joint movement beyond the normal limits.
Individualization	Training according to the abilities and goals of an individual.
Interval training	Training with short periods of high intensity work interspersed with periods of low intensity work.

Isokinetic	With constant speed (rate of change of muscle length).
Isometric	Muscle action without joint movement.
Isotonic	With constant force.
Ligament	A fibrous tissue connecting bones to other bones.
Load	Weight lifted.
Lordosis	Anterior convexity of the spine in the lumbar region. (hyper lordosis is beyond the normal lordosis).
Lumbar	Concerning the lower back.
Oblique curl	Diagonal abdominal curl for the oblique abdominals.
Overload	Training load exceeding the normal magnitude.
Postural	Concerning posture or position.
Power	Work per unit of time (force and speed).
Prophylactic	Preventive (training)
Progressive	Gradual increase, progression.
PROM	Passive Range Of Motion.
Plyometrics	Training method using elastic strength and explosiveness, e.g. jumps and throws.
Push-up	Arm exercise, plank position, bend and extend the arms.
Recovery	Rest period (for improved performance).
Repetition	The number of times an exercise is repeated.
ROM	Range Of Motion, amplitude.
Rotation	Circular movement around a center of rotation, rotation axis; spine right and left rotation, limbs internal and external rotation.
RPE	Rating of Perceived Exertion.
Rest-pause	A short break between sets for recovery.
Sagittal plane	Vertical plane, which passes from front (ventral) to back (rear/dorsal). Forward and backward movement.
SAID principle	Specific Adaptions to Imposed Demand.
Set	A number of repetitions in a series without a rest-pause.
Tendon	A fibrous tissue connecting muscle to bone.
Transverse plane	Horizontal plane, that divides the body into superior and inferior parts. Movement in the horizontal plane.
Weight	The resistance due to gravity.
Work	Force times distance.
Workout	Training session.

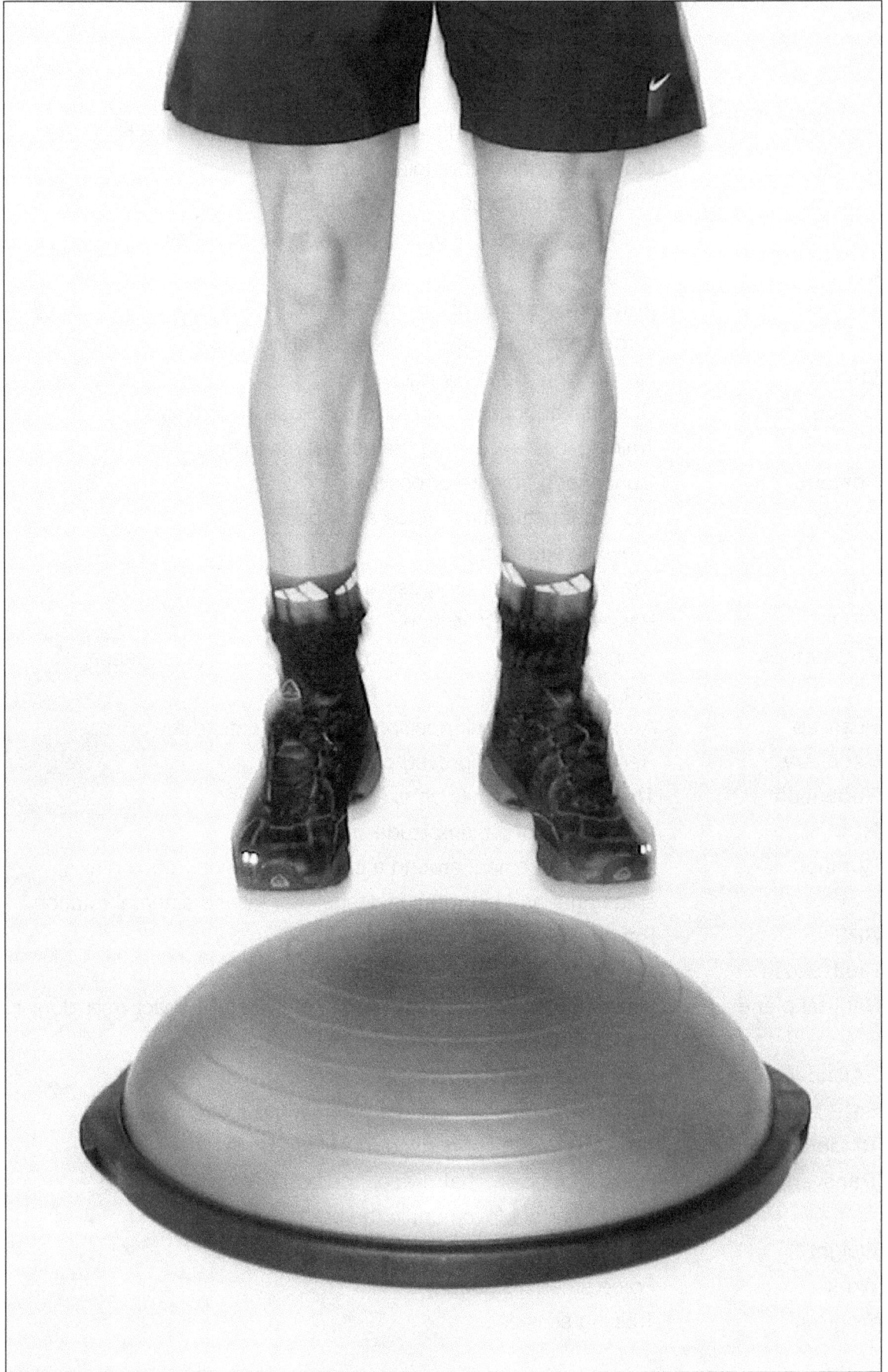

APPENDIX | BOSU TBX and SCX

This book presents two program examples: a verse/chorus concept program BOSU **TBX, Total Body Crosstraining** and a **SCX, Strength and Core Crosstraining** program.

The SCX and TBX programs are for intermediate level exercisers and requires some prior BOSU training. Both programs, however, can easily be adapted for beginners.

The TBX program is an allround workout for improving cardiovascular fitness, coordination, balance, strength and flexibility.

Before starting: The BOSU TBX and BOSU SCX are for healthy exercisers. Get instructions from an experienced trainer or instructor the first couple of BOSU-workouts.

The BOSU can be used for rehabilitation, but this should be supervised by a (physio)therapist.

Abbreviations:

R	Right
L	Left
U	Up
D	Down
I	In
O	Out
F	Forward/front
B	Backward/back
OT	Over the top
ST	Step touch
V	Verse (A-part)
C	Chorus | refrain (B-part)
M	Bridge, transition (C-part)

TBX is choreographed to: MoveYa: Bodystyling House Classics 89-94.

Recommended SCX music, eg. world music (drums), 110-130 BPM.

BOSU TBX

Music time	Part Beats	Technique | tips	Exercise
	Warm-up I 4 x 8 4 x 8 4 x 8	Focus on breath: Inhale (8)/exhale (8) x 2 Tap R/L toes on top, 8 x (HV) Walk 8, 4 x, shake the head, shake arms	
	2 x 8 (piano)	Walk around the BOSU 8, walk 8	
	2 x 8 (0:53) C	Walk slowly **R** UUDD on the BOSU, **2 x**	
	2 x 8 (piano)	Walk around the BOSU 8, walk 8	
	2 x 8 (1:10) V 2 x 8 2 x 8	Walk slowly **R** UUDD on the BOSU, **4 x** Squat (D 2, U 2), 4 x	
Track # 1 (intro)	2 x 8 (1:33) C	Walk slowly **L** UUDD on the BOSU, **2 x**	
Track # 2	2 x 8 (1:40) V 2 x 8	Walk slowly **L** UUDD on the BOSU, **4 x**	
03:43	2 x 8	Squat (D 2, U 2), 4 x (D/U onto toes)	
03:43	2 x 8 (2:04) C	Walk tempo R UUDD on the BOSU 4 x	
Always There	2 x 8	R Mambo UDDD, 4 x	
	2 x 8	L Long mambo, 2 x (forward off BOSU)	
124 BPM	4 x 8	Sidelunge R L (O/I), 2 x 8 x	
	4 x 8	Sidelunge R L (half tempo), 8 x	
	2 x 8 (piano)	Squat (D 2/U 2), 4 x	
	2 x 8 C	Walk tempo L UUDD on the BOSU 4 x	
	2 x 8	L Mambo UDDD, 4 x	
	2 x 8	L Long mambo, 2 x	
	4 x 8	Squat (D 2/U 2), 8 x	

BOSU TBX

Music time	Part Beats	Technique | tips	Exercise
	Warm up II		
	4 x 8	Walk on the floor 8, 4 x	
	4 x 8 (0:15) C	Walk on the top 8, 4 x (step down on count '31', '32')	
	4 x 8 (0:31) V	Skip (4/travel 4) 8	
	4 x 8 (0:46) V	Kneelift (4/travel 4) 8	
	4 x 8 (1:02) C	Walk on the top 8, 4 x (step down on count '31', '32')	
	4 x 8 (1:17) M	Abduction (4/travel 4) 8	
	4 x 8 (1:33) M	Hamstring curl (4/travel 4) 8	
Track # 3 03:36 07:19	4 x 8 (1:49) V	Extension (4/travel 4) 8	
	4 x 8 (2:04) C	Walk on the top 8, 4 x (step down on count '31', '32')	
Gypsy Woman	4 x 8 (2:19) M	Kneelift repeater (3), H	
		Kneelift repeater (3), V	
		Abduction repeater (3), H	
124 BPM		Hamstring curl repeater (3), V	
	4 x 8 (2:31) M	Knee/side/back repeater (3), H, V, H, V	
	4 x 8 (2:51) C	Walk on the top 8, 4 x (step down on count '31', '32')	
	4 x 8 (3:06) M	Knee/side/back repeater (3), H V H V	
	4 x 8 (3:21)	Walk on the floor 8, 4 x	

BOSU TBX

Music time	Part Beats	Technique | tips	Exercise
	Cardio part I		
	4 x 8	Tap R/L on top, 8 x tempo, 4 x half time	
	4 x 8 (0:16) C	Lunge R/L up on the top, 8	
	4 x 8 (0:31) V	Skip 8	
	4 x 8 (0:47) V	L-skip (3) R, L, R, L	
	4 x 8 (1:02) C	Lunge R/L up on the top, 8	
	4 x 8 (1:18) V	(Hip) Extension 8	
Track # 4	4 x 8 (1:33) V	L-extension (3) R, L, R, L	
04:07			
11:26	4 x 8 (1:49) C	Lunge R/L up on the top. 8	
Express Yourself	4 x 8 (2:05) M	Walk on the top 8, 4 x	
124 BPM	4 x 8 (2:20) M	Jog on the top 8, 4 x	
	4 x 8 (2:35) C	Lunge R/L up on the top. 8	
	4 x 8 (2:51) V	L-skip (3) R, L, R, L	
	4 x 8 (3:07) C	Lunge R/L up on the top. 8	
	4 x 8 (3:22) V	L-extension (3) R, L, R, L	
	4 x 8 (3:38) 4 x 8	Lunge F/B/F (hip/hamstring/hip stretch) R 8, L, 8	

BOSU TBX

Music time	Part Beats	Technique | tips	Exercise
Track # 5 04:43 26:09 **The Best Things in Life Are Free** **124 BPM**	Cardio part II 4 x 8	Tap on top RL, 8 x	
	4 x 8 (0:15) V	Step Up, Tap, D, D, R L, 8 x	
	4 x 8 (0:30) V	Step Up Tap DD (sync. hop), RL, 8	
	4 x 8 (0:47) V	Tripple jog on the top, R L, 8 x	
	4 x 8 (1:02) C	Kick 8 (U kick DD)	
	4 x 8 (1:17) M	Chasse R L Kick back R L on floor. Chasse L R Kick back L R on floor, 4 x	
	4 x 8 (1:33) V	Step Up Tap DD (sync. hop), RL, 8	
	4 x 8 (1:49) V	Tripple jog on the top, R L, 8 x	
	4 x 8 (2:04) C	Kick 8 (U kick DD), 1/1 R on BOSU	
	4 x 8 (2:20) C	Kick 8 (U kick DD), 1/1 L on BOSU	
	4 x 8 (2:35) M 2 x 8 (2:50) M	Chasse RL, Kick back, repeat LR, 6 x	
	4 x 8 (2:58) V	Tripple jog on the top, R L, 8 x	
	4 x 8 (3:13) C	Kick 8 (U kick DD), 1/1 R on BOSU	
	4 x 8 (3:29) C	Kick 8 (U kick DD), 1/1 L on BOSU	
	4 x 8 (3:44)	U Tap DD, R L, 8 x	
	4 x 8 (3:59)	U Tap, Down Tap, R L, 8 x	
	2 x 8 (4:15)	Step touch R/L on the floor, 8 On the last one: Go to the right side of the BOSU. Ready to go over the top (left).	

BOSU TBX			
Music time	Part Beats	Technique | tips	Exercise
	Cardio part III		
	4 x 8 (0:08)	Over the top, OT, 8 x	
	4 x 8 (0:16)	Over the top, OT, 8 x	
	4 x 8 (0:31) V	Over the top, OT, power, 8 x	
	4 x 8 (0:47) C	OT, squat on the floor, 4 x	
	4 x 8 (1:01) C	OT, sidelunge on the floor, 4 x	
	4 x 8 (1:17) C	OT, jack 2 on the floor, 4 x	
Track # 6 03:36 29:45	4 x 8 (1:33) V	OT power, 8 x	
	4 x 8 (1:48) C	Step tap sideways up/DD and OT, 4 x	
Finally	4 x 8 (2:04) C	Jump sideways U/hold/DD, OT, 4 x	
124 BPM	4 x 8 (2:20) C	Jump sideways U/jump/DD, OT, 4 x	
	4 x 8 (2:35) V/C	OT power, 8 x	
	4 x 8 (2:50) 'C'	OT – 4 double tempo run/DD, 8 x	
	4 x 8 (3:06) 'C'	OT – 4 double tempo run/DD, 8 x	
	4 x 8 (3:20)	Over the top 4 x	
		Step touch on the floor 2 x + ready (8)	

BOSU TBX

Music time	Part Beats	Technique | tips	Exercise
	Cardio part IV		
	4 x 8	Basic step R (UUDD), 8 x	
	4 x 8 (0:15)	Step up, squat, step down squat, 4 x (UU, Squat D/U, DD, Squat D/U)	
	4 x 8 (0:30) V	UU Lunge/lunge DD, 4 x	
	4 x 8 (0:46) V	UU Lunge while turning 1/1, 2 x	
	4 x 8 (1:02) V	Lunge, 1/1 opposite way, 2 x – DD	
Track # 7	4 x 8 (1:17) C	Basic jog R UUDD, 8 x	
03:52			
33:37	4 x 8 (1:33) M	Step up, squat, step down squat, 4 x (UU, Squat D/U, DD, Squat D/U)	
Show Me Love	4 x 8 (1:49) V	UU Jump 2 (half time) on top DD, 4 x	
	4 x 8 (2:04) V	UU Jump while turning 1/1, 2 x	
124 BPM	4 x 8 (2:20) V	UU Jump 1/1 opposite way, 2 x – DD	
	4 x 8 (2:35) C	Basic run L UUDD, 8 x	
	4 x 8 (2:50) M	Basic step L UUDD, 8 x, move 1/1	
	4 x 8 (3:06) M	Basic step L UUDD, 8 x, opposite way	
	4 x 8 (3:21) O/I	Basic step L/walk 8, 4 x,	
	4 x 8 (3:37) I	Squat 8	

BOSU TBX

Music time	Part Beats	Technique | tips	Exercise
	Cooldown Strength I		
	4 x 8	Kick 4, abduction (side out) 4	
	2 x 8 (0:15)	(Hip) Extension 4	
	4 x 8 (0:23) V	Kick slow H V, abduction slow R L	
	4 x 8 (0:39) V	Extension slow R L R L	
	2 x 8 (0:54) M	Walk on the top 8, 2 x	
	4 x 8 (1:01) V	Lunge backward R L, 8 x	
Track # 8	4 x 8 (1:17) C	Squat w/rotation D4/U4 (R L) 8 x	
03:52	4 x 8 (1:33) V		
37:29	4 x 8 (1:48) M	Walk on the top, eg. 4 x	
A Deeper Love	2 x 8 (2:04) M	Walk in front of the BOSU on the floor 8, 2 x	
	2 x 8 (2:11) C	Squat (D2/U2), 4 x	
124 BPM	4 x 8 (2:19) V	Bulgarian lunge R D/U (1-4), 8 x	
	4 x 8 (2:35) V	Bulgarian lunge L R/U (1-4), 8 x	
		Step up (backward, be careful) or: R and L foot step out, out to R and L of BOSU. From there step up.	
	4 x 8 (2:50) C	Squat w/rotation D4/U4 (R L) 8 x	
	4 x 8 (3:05) C		
	4 x 8 (3:20)	Walk, on the top 8, 4 x	
	4 x 8 (3:35)	Walk on the floor 8, 4 x Let the hands slide down the legs. Put the hands on the BOSU. Walk back with the feet. Ready.	

BOSU TBX

Music time	Part Beats	Technique | tips	Exercise
	Strength II		
	2 x 8	Push-ups, D/U (down 1-4, up 5-8), 2	
	2 x 8 (0:08)	T-push-up, (bend, extend and rotate)	
	2 x 8 (0:16)	RL, 4	
	4 x 8 (0:23)	T-push-up, RL, 4	
	4 x 8 (0:39)	Back extension (kneeling), 4 x	
	4 x 8 (0:54) C	Back extension with back fly, 4 x	
Track # 9	2 x 8 (1:10) M	Sit back, easy stretch, turn the BOSU.	
03:21	4 x 8 (1:19) V	Push-ups, wide, 8	
40:50	4 x 8 (1:33) V		
	4 x 8 (1:48) M	Sit back easy stretch, turn the BOSU.	
Groove Is In the Heart	4 x 8 (2:04) C	Back extension with back fly, 4 x	
124 BPM	4 x 8 (2:19) M	Stretch, cat-camel, 4 x	
	4 x 8 (2:34) C	Back extension with back fly, 4 x	
	4 x 8 (2:50) M	Stretch, cat-camel, 4 x	
	4 x 8 (3:06)	Balance on all fous Move the hips to the side. R L R L.	

BOSU TBX

Music time	Part Beats	Technique | tips	Exercise
	Strength III		
	2 x 8	Check the technique, stabilize.	
	2 x 8 (0:08)	Neck and spine in neutral position.	
	2 x 8 (0:16)	Lift hand and opposite knee, alternate.	
	4 x 8 (0:22) V	Alternating superman 8	
	4 x 8 (0:39) V		
	4 x 8 (0:54) C	Prone back extension 4	
	4 x 8 (1:10) M	Prone back extension 4	
		(or transition to the left side)	
Track # 10	4 x 8 (1:25) V	Sidebend (curl), R (legs to the side), 8	
03:44	4 x 8 (1:40) V		
44:34	4 x 8 (1:56) C	Ab curl 8	
Hold On Tighter	4 x 8 (2:12) M	Bridge, dynamic, 4	
	4 x 8 (2:27) M	Bridge, dynamic, 4	
		(or transition to the L)	
	4 x 8 (2:43) C	Sidebend (curl), L (legs to the side), 8	
	4 x 8 (2:58) C		
	4 x 8 (3:13) M	Ab curl 8	
	4 x 8 (3:29)	Roll up 8, Stand up 8, Walk 8, Walk back to starting position 8	
	Fade music ... Forward to track #19		

BOSU TBX

Music time	Part Beats	Technique | tips	Exercise
Track # 19 04:02 48:36 **Keep On Moving** **90 BPM**	Stretching I 2 x 8 stretching 1 x 8 transition	Stretch: Hip flexors Calves, straight and bent knee Thighs Hamstrings Adductors, one side Adductors, other side Abductors Buttocks Repeat, opposite leg leads	
Track # 20 03:50 52:26 **Nothing Com-pares 2 U** **0 BPM**	Stretching II 2 x 8 / stretching 1 x 8 / transition	Stand in front of the BOSU, rolll D/U 2 (4) x. Sit on the BOSU after the last one. Triceps stretch (back of the arm). Shoulder, posterior part. Shoulder, medial part. Repeat opposite. Then arms out (chest stretch) Legs in front, 'sandwich' stretch Bend the legs, legs (knees) out, adductor stretch Sidebend R, sidebend L. Legs together and stand op. Rotate and shake it out.	

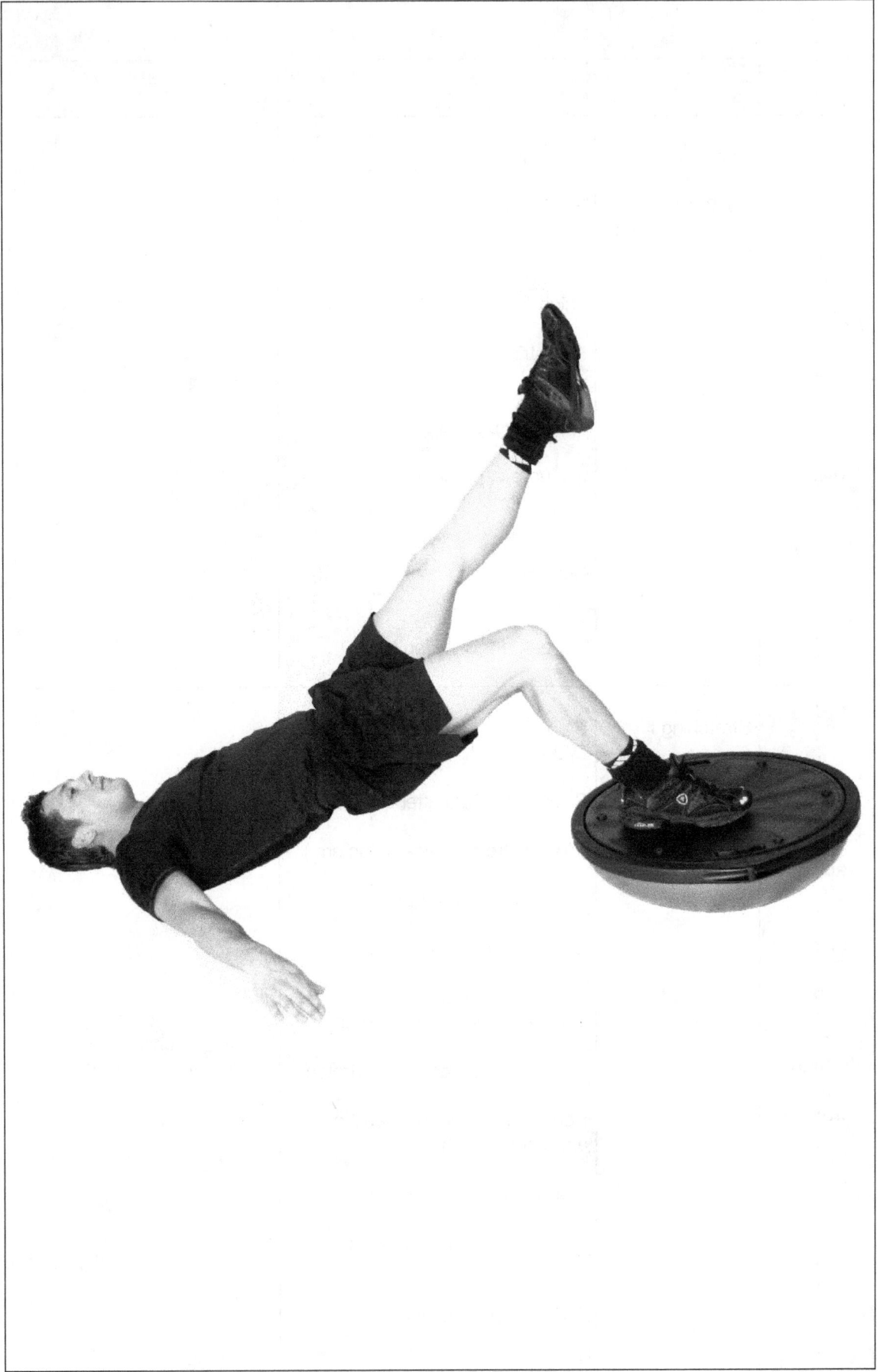

BOSU SCX

Sets Repetitions	Exercise
7-10 min.	Warm-up with dynamic, low-impact movements
Dynamic exercises: 1-3 sets 8-12 repetitions	Lunge back from the top Parallel squat lunge > Squat side lunge, kneelift, reverse lunge, kneeligt, squat side lunge, kneelift Squat w/rotation Overhead lunge (from floor to top) Deadlift with BOSU (or 'swing' BOSU) Push-ups, hands on the BOSU, walkout push-ups (feet on the BOSU) Rowing with the BOSU (unilateral rowing)
Isometric exercises 1-3 sets 15-120 seconds	Asymmetrical plank Alternating superman Back extension Turning torso (plank 4 x 1/4 turn) (on hands or forearms) Supine dying bug (unilateral arm/leg drop) Leg drops (as variation) Bridge, dynamic, on one leg, right and left Ab curl, one bent, one straight leg, hand-to-foot, right and left (BOSU test)
5-10 min.	Cool-down with stretching

ABOUT THE AUTHOR

Marina Aagaard, Master of Fitness and Exercise, part-time associate professor of sports (fitness/dance) and guest lecturer at the Academy of Coaching and Tradium.

She is former national coach of AER gymnastics and consultant and course instructor for the Danish Gymnastics Federation and Sports Confederation of Denmark in charge of education, conventions and development from 1995-2008.

Before that, Marina was regional manager of aerobics and club manager for the health club chain Form og Figur, 1990-1991, and managing director of the family health club BodyTeria, 1991-1999.

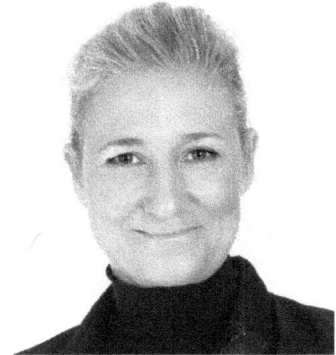

At the same time Marina have been busy as a consultant at her own company aagaard as an advisor and lecturer for many different organisations.

Marina has enjoyed strength training and group exercise since 1983 and, starting, 1987 she has written numerous artcles on health and fitness for newspapers and magazines. She is the author of a bestselling series of fitness books.

Marina is a certified Holistic Lifestyle Coach, CHEK Institute, as well as a certified aerobics instructor and personal trainer (gold), American Council on Exercise.

During the 90's she managed the Danish Reebok Instructor Club and worked as Master Trainer, Step og Slide Reebok. In 1993-1994 she starred in the Eurosports Step Reebok serie together with Gin Miller, the inventor of step training.

Later on Marina had her own morning-TV fitness show for a two year period at local television.
As a choreographer Marina created several shows for national television, DR, dance and fitness programmes.

Marinas interest for elite training and performance lead to judging activity within the IAF, NAC, FISAF and the first Miss Fitness competitions in Denmark. Marina went on to serve as a juge breveté, a.o. difficulty judge, in AER gymnastics for the Federation Internationale de Gymnastique, FIG, and served as a judge at every EC, WC and World Series final from 1995-2003.

Marina lives with her husband architect Henrik Elstrup in the bay area of Kaloe Vig in Jutland, Denmark. Her interests are fitness and wellness, running, skiing and skating, arts, music, dance, nature, travelling and cars.

FITNESS BOOKS

Stability Ball Exercises
Fitness and Performance Exercises for
Strength, Stability and Flexibility
274 pages

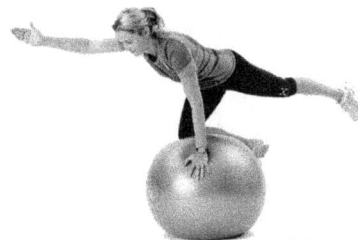

A comprehensive compilation of stability ball
exercises. Over 450 exercises with the stability
ball, also know as the Swiss ball or strength ball.
Plus even more variations.
One-on-one, partner and group exercises at all
levels, for beginners, intermediate and advanced
exercisers, including Olympic Athletes.
With more than 900 photos and step-by-step
text on proper exercise technique. And a guide
to progressing ball exercises.
As a unique feature the book includes the most
effective and enjoyable warm-up/cardio and
stretching exercises with the ball.
Stability Ball Exercises, a Scandinavian bestseller,
is a valuable reference book for any coach, trainer,
physical exercise leader, personal trainer, group
exercise instructor, physiotherapist and PE teacher.

**STABILITY BALL
EXERCISES**

Fitness and Performance Exercises
for Strength, Stability and Flexibily

Scandinavian
Bestseller
450 Exercises for Trainers,
PE Teachers, Therapists
and Exercisers

Marina Aagaard, MFE

Resistance Training Exercises
Fitness and Performance Exercises for
Strength, Stability and Mobility
290 pages

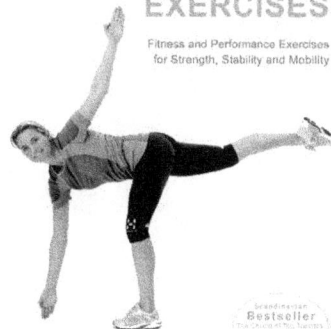

A comprehensive compilation of resistance
training exercises. Over 500 exercises; bodyweight,
dumbbells, barbells, tubes, bands and balls.
For one-on-one, partner and group strength training
at all levels, beginners, intermediate and advanced.
With more than 1000 photos and step-by-step
text on proper exercise technique, basic posture,
starting position and safety precautions.
The book features basic, intermediate as well as
advanced exercises from top to toe, from inner
unit to outer unit, for optimal health, fitness and
performance and enjoyable, time-efficient workouts.
Including a comprehensive partner exercise section.
Resistance Training Exercises, a Scandinavian
bestseller, is a valuable reference book for any
coach, trainer, physical exercise leader, personal
trainer, fitness instructor, group exercise instructor,
physiotherapist and PE teacher.

**RESISTANCE
TRAINING
EXERCISES**

Fitness and Performance Exercises
for Strength, Stability and Mobility

Scandinavian
bestseller

Marina Aagaard, MFE

www.ingramcontent.com/pod-product-compliance
Lightning Source LLC
Chambersburg PA
CBHW080852300326
41935CB00041B/1553